The Immunology of Infant Feeding

ETTORE MAJORANA INTERNATIONAL SCIENCE SERIES

Series Editor:

Antonino Zichichi
European Physical Society
Geneva, Switzerland

(LIFE SCIENCES)

The Immunology of Infant Feeding

Edited by

A. W. Wilkinson

Institute of Child Health
University of London
London, England

PLENUM PRESS · NEW YORK AND LONDON

Library of Congress Cataloging in Publication Data

International School of Medical Sciences (13th : 1980 : Erice, Italy)
   The immunology of infant feeding.

   (Ettore Majorana international science series. Life sciences ; 8)
   ''Proceedings of the 13th course of the International School of Medical
Sciences, held September 21-28, 1980, the Ettore Majorana Center for Scientific
Culture, Erice, Sicily, Italy.''—Verso of t.p.
   Bibliography: p.
   Includes index.
   1. Infants—Nutrition—Immunological aspects—Congress. 2. Breast feeding—
Immunological aspects—Congresses. 3. Malnutrition in children—Immunological
aspects—Congresses. 4. Immunologic diseases in children—Nutritional aspects—
Congresses. I. Wilkinson, A. W. (Andrew Wood). II. Title. III. Series. [DNLM: 1.
Allergy and immunology—Congresses. 2. Infant nutrition—Congresses.
W1 ET712M v. 8 / WS 120 I61i 1980]

RJ216.I56 1980	613.2'6'0880542	81-10736
ISBN-13: 978-1-4684-4051-5	e-ISBN-13: 978-1-4684-4049-2	AACR2
DOI: 10.1007/978-1-4684-4049-2		

Proceedings of the 13th Course of the International School
of Medical Sciences, held September 21-28, 1980, at the
Ettore Majorana Center for Scientific Culture, Erice,
Sicily, Italy

FOREWORD

    Though much thought is given to nutritional aspects of infant
feeding, the complex immunological aspects have not been considered
adequately, not only in the acceptance of the change to artificial
feeding during this century, but also in developing feeds for total
or supplementary feeding which will do minimal immunological damage.

    Besides food, mother's milk gives an orchestra of complex
interacting bacteriostatic, bactericidal and anti-viral substances
which contribute to the establishment of the normal intestinal flora.
These mechanisms probably explain the many reports that breast fed
babies get fewer infections than those fed artificially; deprivation
from this effect of artificial feeding can be devastating in
developing countries, with limited hygienic facilities, bad water
supplies and sanitation. Infection is also more frequent in
artificially fed infants in developed countries.

    Ingesting antigens is an important step in initiating the immune
response, but the response to such antigens is a controlled one,
and besides antibody and cell mediated responses, partial tolerance,
and immune exclusion (reduction of subsequent entry of antigen)
occur. It is likely that food allergy, grossly neglected until
recently, arises from disturbance of such mechanisms in the
genetically vulnerable (immunodeficient) child.

    The role of such common minor genetic heterogeneity on the risk
of infection resulting from artificial feeding has been little
studied. The development of atopic allergies is strongly influenced
by adverse environmental factors in the neonatal period, one of which
is infant feeding. In this book we consider mechanisms and genetic
variation in response to, and the handling of ingested antigen, the
mechanisms of protection transferred by the mother, the nature of
the intestinal flora and the way in which artificial feeding and
supplements affect it. The possibility that such changes in
intestinal flora affect chronic immunopathology is also considered.

It is also important, for immunological as well as other
reasons, for the infant to have enough to eat. The adverse effects
of malnutrition on antibody and cell mediated immune responses are
also outlined, with recognition of the importance of the deterioration
of infectious illness which accompanies weaning in developing
countries, in the development of the syndromes of malnutrition.
Finally, the implications of these factors for planning immunisation,
milk banks, and artificial feeds are considered, and in particular
whether feeds to supplement breast feeding should differ from those
for total infant feeding. Finally suggestions are made for further
fields requiring more study, and longer term and immediate research
possibilities.

The principal deduction from the fruitful discussion at this
lively meeting was the profound limitation of our knowledge of all
aspects of this complex field. Nonetheless, there is plenty of
evidence for the complexity of these inter-relationships, and the
abandoning or supplementation of breast feeding is associated with
some increased risk in all countries. The pressing need to prevent
the spread of unnecessarily artificial feeding in developing
communities, should not deflect us from awareness of our ignorance
of the effect such changes may have had in developed countries.
Immunological theory can suggest that many adverse effects, early
and late, may arise from deprivation or inactivation of maternal
protective systems, perhaps especially in some vulnerable individuals.
The only rational deduction is that such a physiological system
should be left undisturbed, unless unavoidable, until we know for
certain that it is safe to do so.

J.F. Soothill

CONTENTS

THE SECRETORY IMMUNE SYSTEM

John Bienenstock[†]

Host Resistance Programme & Department of Pathology
McMaster University Health Sciences Centre
Hamilton, Ontario, Canada

When we consider that we interact with our environment and are
separated from it by only a thin layer of cells, it is not surprising
that an immune system has evolved to regulate potentially pathogenic
organisms and products of that environment such as dietary antigens.
It is my purpose briefly to review the secretory or mucosal immune
system and attempt to show how far this system is integrated with the
rest of the immunologic apparatus. The material contained in this
contribution may be found in an expanded form elsewhere[1,2].

SECRETION IMMUNOGLOBULINS

From an immunological point of view external secretions are
characterised by the presence of the secretory IgA (sIgA) immunoglobulin class. IgA is only one component of the mucosal immune
response and although this molecule remains a marker of that response,
cellular and other humoral mechanisms must also be considered in any
assessment of mucosal resistance.

The secretory IgA molecule is in a special dimeric form and
contains two extra polypeptides known as J chain and secretory component[3]. The J chain is synthesised in plasma cells in the lamina
propria lying beneath the basement membrane of the epithelial cell
layer. The secretory component is synthesised and secreted by serous
glandular epithelial cells. The transport of the dimeric IgA across
the mucosal epithelial layer occurs by covalent interaction with the
secretory component at the lateral and basal portion of the cell
membrane. After incorporation into vesicles the molecules are trans-

---

[†]Supported by the Medical Research Council of Canada

ported across the cells and secreted into the lumen by exocytosis.
The sIgA is incorporated into mucus and possibly covalently bound
to mucin. In IgA deficiency states IgM replaces IgA both in the
cellular content of the lamina propria and also the humoral content
of the secretions. In the secretions IgM is non-covalently bound
to secretory component and shares the same transport pathway as IgA.
Human SC has approximately equal affinity for IgA and IgM.

IgE may also be considered as a true mucosal antibody and much
is synthesised locally in the mucosal tissues of the gastrointestinal and respiratory tracts. This molecule does not complex
to secretory component and is found only in selected groups of
secretions. It is not found in breast milk.

Although the majority of dimeric IgA may be locally synthesised
and secreted on to the local mucosal epithelial surface some is also
found in the lymphatics which drain mucosal tissues. Dimeric IgA
has been shown[4,5] to have a selective transport advantage across
the hepatic parenchymal cell and this appears to be dependent upon
the expression of secretory component on this cell surface, certainly
in the rat and maybe also in the human. Monomeric and sIgA are not
transported by the hepatic parenchymal cells in a selective
fashion[6]. It is not known whether a similar selective transport
system exists for IgM. This selective IgA transport system probably
exists also in most mucosal glandular tissues and such a system occurs
in the salivary gland[7] and the breast[8]. It seems likely that a
similar system will be shown to exist in all tissues where secretory
component is synthesised.

It may be concluded that the presence of sIgA in a particular
external secretion may indicate local synthesis and local secretion
by lymphocytes in the local mucosal tissue. However local synthesis
with distant secretion may also have occurred. The exact extent to
which this transport system exists in glandular mucosal tissues other
than the breast, salivary gland and gastrointestinal tract is not
known and awaits definition.

Function of secretory IgA

The sIgA is resistant to proteolysis, prevents adherence and
colonisation of bacteria on epithelial surfaces, may block complement
fixation by complement fixing antibodies, acts as a blocking antibody in hypersensitivity reactions and may also exclude macromolecular
uptake by both GI and respiratory tracts (immune exclusion). The
possible role of IgA in the regulation of dietary antigen access
across the intestinal mucosal epithelium to the internal milieu has
been the subject of extensive work[9]. The importance of this for
control of antigen access both for the local and systemic immune
systems may be of crucial significance to the subsequent development
of allergy to environmental antigens.

Speculations on the role of IgA

      Although in the past much emphasis has been placed on the role
of the IgA molecule in defence against potential pathogens it may
have a greater and more biologically significant role in the regulation of antigen access to the systemic circulation. Much of the
IgA locally synthesised is directed against dietary antigens. It is
tempting to speculate that dimeric IgA immune complexes of limited
size would share the selective transport advantage which is found
particularly in the liver. Thus dietary and other antigens complexed
to dimeric IgA, synthesised largely in the intestine, would be
selectively cleared from the circulation, not necessarily by the
reticuloendothelial system, but by the hepatic parenchymal cells,
capable of detoxification of a wide variety of potentially toxic
agents. Their secretion into the bile would still retain an
additional potential advantage since they could be further degraded
in the intestinal lumen and be utilised as a source of nutrition.
Furthermore this might allow the mucosal immune system "a second
chance" to process the material as antigen for a local mucosal immune
response. The selective IgA transport system in glands might also
account for the antigenic drive for proliferation of mucosal lymphocytes in tissues such as the salivary gland and the breast, generally
considered to be sterile and thus without obvious drive.

      In this way mucosa associated lymphoid tissue (MALT) derived
lymphocytes would have seeded these tissues and the presence of
dimeric IgA packaged to antigen encountered in the intestine might
provide an additional proliferative drive for the retention of such
cells locally in salivary glands. Antigen administered intravenously
may be selectively secreted into the milk of lactating mothers and
may even cause the induction of immunologic tolerance in suckling
neonates by the absorption of the tolerogen through the gastrointestinal tract[10]. Further the intestinal absorption of immune
complexes by neonatal rats is the means whereby increased antigen
uptake may occur accross the intestinal epithelium before closure
occurs[11]. It seems likely that the presence of IgA immune complexes
in the intestinal lumen of the offspring may be expected to be
involved in the regulation of the subsequent immune response. It
has been suggested that after oral immunisation circulating IgA
immune complexes may be tolerogenic[12] but this has not been confirmed. Indeed such IgA immune complexes are rapidly cleared from
the circulation and even act as a primer for a subsequent IgG and IgM
response[13]. Furthermore polymorphonuclear leukocytes appear to
possess IgA receptors and the extent to which macrophages may
similarly possess such receptors for dimeric IgA is unknown at
present, although it may even provide for macrophages derived from
mucosal tissues with putative IgA receptors on their cell surface,
a means whereby they might be retained in mucosal tissues.

This hypothesis is attractive since it may offer an explanation for the maintenance of the proliferative drive of IgA producing cells in mucosal sites normally not exposed to antigenic stimulation. Furthermore it may also offer a more significant reason for the presence of IgA in mucosal tissues. If this is accepted then the purported defence mechanisms mediated by the secretory IgA molecule at mucosal surfaces may be secondary in importance to the one just outlined.

MUCOSAL LYMPHOID TISSUE AND THE TRAFFIC OF LYMPHOID CELLS

B blasts

Two types of lymphoid aggregates are found in mammalian intestine. The first consists of multiple aggregates and is known as Peyer's patches. The second consists of isolated lymphoid follicles scattered throughout the intestine and often prominent in the colon. These have been termed solitary lymphoid nodules (SLN). Similar collections of lymphoid aggregates of both types of morphology exist in the bronchial mucosa[14,15]. Both types of aggregates possess a specialised lymphoepithelium termed M cells which possess the capacity selectively to concentrate antigen especially from the luminal side. This lymphoepithelium is very similar to that found over the dome of bursal follicles in the chicken.

Such mucosal follicles may also exist in other glandular tissues and Ham[16] has described the SLN as being characteristic of wet mucosal epithelial membranes. In any event they may be grouped together and termed MALT. Cells derived from the gut and bronchus associated lymphoid tissue (GALT and BALT) have been shown several days after transfer into lethally irradiated rabbits to contain predominantly IgA[17]. Lymphoblasts from the mesenteric lymph node or thoracic duct have a selective localisation potential for the small intestine[18] and such blast cells after transfer in a syngenic system are localised primarily in the small intestine although a half to a third as many are found in the colon. In both sites these newly localised cells predominantly contain IgA. The Peyer's patches contain a population of precursor cells bearing IgA which migrate via the mesenteric lymph node the the thoracic duct and are then found in peripheral mucosal sites making IgA[19]. Peripheral sites which have been identified in this IgA localisation route include the mammary gland, the bronchus, the salivary gland and breast[19,20,21]. It is still uncertain which other mucosal and glandular tissues belong to this common mucosal immune system[22].

Goldblum et al.[23] showed specific IgA antibody and specific IgA antibody containing cells capable of activity in a plaque assay in the milk of lactating human females who had been fed non-pathogenic E. coli. The localisation of such cells in the mammary glands and cervix appears to be under the influence of sex hormones[24,25]. B blasts derived from the bronchial lymph node and found subsequently in the bronchus and intestine synthesise IgA. Such cells derived from the lung have a marked tendency to return to the lung but those derived from the mesenteric node selectively repopulate the intestine. Thus the organ of source appears to be an important factor in determining the subsequent destination.

Two models might be considered which would account for this type of localisation. The first would suggest that lymphocyte surface characteristics with complementary receptors, expressed within the vascular compartment in mucosal tissues, might be responsible for the emigration of cells in these sites. This appears unlikely since removal of Peyer's patches in experimental rats did not affect the localisation of blasts in the intestine[26]. Peyer's patches are the only sites in the intestine at which there are post-capillary venules which are known to transmit small lymphocytes and blast cells. The second possibility is that there might be a random migration of blasts from the vascular compartment with selective retention by at present unknown factors in the tissues. This is more attractive but more difficult to define and the lengthy list of such possible factors includes secretory component, hormone and antigen receptors, chemo-tactic factor receptors, and receptors for T helper cell products. Blood flow also appears to be important. Although antigen amplifies the localisation of primed mucosal IgA precursors[27], such cells localise in the intestines of germ-free animals, in foetal intestine and in lung transplanted under the capsule of a kidney subcutaneously. Thus antigen is not essential for the localisation of these cells in mucosal tissues.

Peyer's patches have the potential to repopulate the immune system with cells other than those which contain IgA immunoglobulin. A single shielded Peyer's patch can repopulate the entire lymphoid tissues of an irradiated animal[28]. MLN compared with peripheral nodes is a major source of intestinal IgG and IgM precursor cells[19]; thirteen times as many cells containing IgG are found in the intestine after MLN transfer than after PLN or BLN, whereas twelve times as many cells containing IgG were found in the lung after transfer of BLN as when peripheral node cells were used as donors. Thus there may even be a selective mucosal localisation for IgG cells.

Studies of IgE synthesis have shown that this immunoglobulin is synthesised by GALT, MLN and BLN[29]. In the Peyer's patches of germ-free rats relatively large numbers of presumed B lymphocytes bearing IgE have been described[30]. Local immunisation of the lung relative to foot pad immunisation led to the appearance of IgE anti-body synthesis locally in the draining bronchial nodes[29]. Although it is therefore possible that cells destined to synthesise IgE may be found predominantly in MALT such as BALT and GALT, the migration, localisation and differentiation of these cells may be controlled by the environment of the upper and lower respiratory tract and

intestine. Since such cells appear to be missing in sex hormone
target tissues such as the breast, sex hormonal influence on the
localisation of such cells in these tissues may be very different
from that on IgA B blasts.

T blasts

T immunoblasts from MLN and TD have a tendency to localise in
lamina propria and also the villous epithelium of both normal adult
GALT as well as in foetal gut isografts. The lymphocytes in the
epithelium are thought to be almost exclusively T cells, have a
different half life than the columnar epithelial cells which migrate
over the top of them, contain metachromatic granules[31], but have
low concentrations of histamine and serotonin[32]. The relationship
of these cells to mucosal lymphocytes in other mucosal tissues such
as the respiratory and urogenital tracts, and mammary glands is not
known.

Oral immunisation may lead to the generation of cytotoxic T
cells in Peyer's patches and in extra-intestinal sites[33]. Administration of antigen to the GI or respiratory tracts leads to the
appearance of cells in these tissues which release macrophage
inhibition factor upon challenge with antigen, but it is not known
whether these cells are T lymphocytes[34,35]. Human milk lymphocytes
respond by proliferation when exposed to antigens expressed at other
mucosal sites particularly those related to enteric flora[36], and
there is circumstantial evidence that T blasts may also have a
tendency, if derived from the gut, to go back to that site. Since
epithelial lymphocytes occupy an inter-epithelial site and this is
in the direct path of antigen which crosses the intestinal epithelium,
if these cells are antigen reactive they may release substances which
may affect the integrity and function of the intestinal epithelium,
and thereby influence local and systemic immunity in a highly
significant fashion.

Macrophages

Following oral feeding antigen may appear in macrophage-like
cells below the basement membrane in the lamina propria of villi.
The GI and respiratory tract epithelia do not serve as a total
barrier to macromolecules or even particulate material. It has been
known for a long time that bacteriophages, viruses and even particulate matter may cross in variable amounts into the systemic
circulation[37]. When latex particles or other materials are fed to
animals they may be found in macrophages in the intestinal lamina
propria. Macrophages are also found in the domes and follicles of
Peyer's patches as well as BALT, and tingible body macrophages have
also been shown there. The specialised lymphoepithelium which contains M cells appears selectively to sample the environment. Despite
this the cells in MALT appear to have a relative or absolute

deficiency in the accessory adherent cells necessary for the expression of a primary immune response in vitro[39]. Since it appears likely that GALT contains cells already primed and that therefore priming does not occur locally in MALT the functional purpose of the M cells may be to cause proliferation of cells already primed[39]. Such macrophages from the intestine do migrate and can be found in thoracic duct lymph after mesenteric adenectomy[40]. It is possible that such macrophages came from Peyer's patches or even the lamina propria. The possibility exists that they may themselves have a selective migration pattern which would influence the subsequent quality of the immune response.

IMMUNISATION AND REGULATION OF IMMUNITY

Positive events

Studies of the appearance of cells containing antibody in thoracic duct lymph and the lamina propria have shown the classical appearance of a hastened response after secondary challenge, especially when the primary challenge was parenteral and the secondary was oral[27]. This discrepancy may be explained if we remember that secretion by plasma cells of the antibody they synthesise might be under separate regulation. It is well known that the functions of synthesis and secretion may be separable as is found in man in the non-secretor myelomas. Thus it would be inappropriate to equate the presence of cells containing antibody with the appearance of antibody in the local secretions.

Very little is known about materials which act as adjuvants for the mucosal immune system, although vitamin A has been shown to have some adjuvant effect (41). In man parenteral immunisation against Cholera toxoid can induce specific IgA antibodies in secretions but this is likely to be due to the previous natural exposure to the vibrio which acted as a priming dose[42]. Similarly it has been possible to immunise against a necrotising enteritis caused by Clostridium welchii through parenteral immunisation[43]. A number of important factors must be considered in any attempt to get the best secretory immune responses. These include previous exposure to the antigen and the dose and route of primer and booster. The concept of the common mucosal immune system and for which considerable evidence now exists, appears to suggest a possible approach. It has been possible to immunise mice by oral vaccination with Herpes type I against intravaginal challenge with Herpes type II[44]. Similar approaches have led to resistance to conjunctival and vaginal challenge to Chlamydia in guinea pigs given a live oral vaccine[45] and immunisation against orally presented antigens has been shown to induce antibodies in milk, lacrymal and salivary secretions.

Negative events

It should be recognised that whenever oral immunisation is under-taken there is a concomitant development of a negative or regulatory immune event. Whenever oral immunisation occurs such a regulatory influence induction is inevitable[46,47]. It is well established that depending on the dose, a variety of orally presented antigens may cause partial or complete tolerance. It is possible that this type of tolerance (the Sulzberger-Chase phenomenon) may not be peculiar to the intestine since the instillation of soluble metal salts into the respiratory tract rendered mice tolerant to subsequent challenge with the specific chemical[48]. The mechanism whereby this regulation and potential suppression of the immune response occurs after mucosal presentation of antigen is highly complicated. T and B suppressor cells, macrophages and the prostaglandins which they synthesise, as well as IgG1 specific for the immunising antigen have all been implicated in mediation of orally induced tolerance[49,50, 51,52]. It is particularly interesting that suppressor cells specific for the IgA class have been shown to be present in sequential order of appearance in GALT followed by mesenteric node and spleen. Furthermore cells specific for the suppression of IgE may also be found in the Peyer's patches of mice receiving oral ovalbumin[53].

ENVIRONMENT

Since we are continually interacting with a heterogeneous group of antigens in the external environment it is not surprising that factors in the diet may influence local immune responses. The products of digestion, such as simple sugars including L-fucose and L-rhamnose, may totally inhibit various lymphocyte activities both in vitro and in vivo[54,55]. Therefore the major processes of digestion itself may have a marked regulatory influence. Endotoxin has been shown to depress the development of cell-mediated cyto-toxicity possibly through lipid A and similarly lipopolysaccharide may provide a microbial induced signal to generate suppressive influences which are remarkably deficient in germ-free animals[56].

Many factors have been described in colostrum and milk which can affect the maturity and numbers of cells containing immuno-globulin; one such factor which may promote IgA synthesis and secretion has been found in human milk[57] and similar factors have been described also in pigs[58], and others may reduce the capacity of the offspring to mount an IgE immune response[59].

Mucosal and systemic immune responses may be expected to be directly affected to a greater or lesser extent by our external environment and an exploration of this area may lead to a much clearer understanding of how the integrity of our mucosal surfaces is maintained. It is to be hoped that this will lead to therapeutic approaches which will enable us to manipulate this information to our advantage.

REFERENCES

1. Bienenstock J. and Befus A.D.M., in Strober W. ed., Humana, N.J.
    (in press).
2. Bienenstock J. and Befus A.D.M., Immunology (in press).
3. Heremans J.F. (1974) in "The Antigens, II", ed. Sela M.,
    Academic PRess, N.Y., p. 365.
4. Lemaitre-Coelho I., Jackson G.D.F. and Vaerman J-P. (1978)
    J. Exp. Med. 147: 934.
5. Orlans E., Peppard J., Reynolds J. and Hall J. (1978) J. Exp.
    Med. 147: 588.
6. Socken D.J. and Underdown B.J. (1978) Immunochemistry 15: 499.
7. Montgomery P.C., Khaleel S.A., Goudswaard J. and Virella G.
    (1977) Immunol. Commun. 6: 683.
8. Halsey J.F., Johnson B.H. and Cebra J.J. (1980) J. Exp. Med.
    151: 767.
9. Walker W.A. and Isselbacher K.J. (1977) New Eng. J. Med. 297:
    767.
10. Halsey J.F. and Benjamin D.C. (1976) J. Immunol. 116: 1204.
11. Abrahamson D.R., Powers A. and Rodewald R. (1979) Science 206:
    567.
12. Ancre C., Heremans J.F., Vaerman J-P. and Cambiaso C.L. (1975)
    J. Exp. Med. 142: 1509.
13. Stokes C.R., Swarbrick E.T. and Soothill J.F. (1980) Immunol.
    40: 455.
14. Bienenstock J, Johnston H. and Perey D.Y.E. (1973) Lab. Invest.
    28: 686.
15. Bienenstock J. Johnston N. and Perey D.Y.E. (1973) Lab. Invest.
    28: 693.
16. Ham A.W. (1969) "Histology" Lipincott, New York, p. 313.
17. Rudzik O., Clancy R.L., Perey D.Y.E., Day R.P. and
    Bienenstock J. (1975) J. Immunol. 114: 1599.
18. Hall J.G. and Smith M.E. (1970) Nature 226: 262.
19. McDermott M.R. and Bienenstock J. (1979) J. Immunol. 122:1892.
20. Weisz-Carrington P., Roux M.E., McWilliams M, Phillips-
    Quagliata J.M. and Lamm M.E. (1979) J. Immunol. 123: 1705.
21. Roux M.E., McWilliams M., Phillips-Quagliata J.M., Weisz-
    Carrington P. and Lamm M.E. (1977) J. Exp. Med. 146: 1311.
22. Bienenstock J. (1974) Prog. Immunol. II, 4:197.
23. Goldblum R.M. Ahlstedt S, Carlsson B., Hanson L.A., Jodal V.,
    Lidin-Janson G. and Sohl-Akerlund A. (1975) Nature 257: 797.
24. Weisz-Carrington P., Roux M.E., McWilliams M., Phillips-
    Quagliata J.M. and Lamm M.E. (1978) Proc. Nat. Acad. Sci.
    USA 75: 2928.
25. McDermott M.R., Clark D.A. and Bienenstock J. (1980) J.
    Immunol. 124: 2536.
26. McDermott M.R., Heatly V., Befus A.D. and Bienenstock H. (1980)
    J. Cell. Immunol. (in press).
27. Pierce N.F. and Gowans J.L. (1975) J. Exp. Med. 142: 1550.

28.   Jacobson L.O., Marks E.K., Simmons E.L. and Gaston E.O. (1961)
          Proc. Soc. Exp. Biol. Med. 108: 487.
29.   Gerbrandy J.L.F. and Bienenstock J. (1976) J. Immunol. 31: 913.
30.   Durkin H.G. and Waksman B.H. (1979) Fed. Proc. 38: 1081.
31.   Ferguson A. (1977) Gut 18: 921.
32.   Guy-Grand D., Griscelli C. and Vassalli P. (1978) J. Exp. Med.
          148: 1661.
33.   Kagnoff M.F. (1978) J. Immunol. 120: 395.
34.   Frederick G.T. and Bohl E.G. (1976) J. Immunol. 116: 1000.
35.   Henney C.S. and Waldmann R.H. (1970) Science 169: 696.
36.   Parmely M.J., Reath D.B., Beer A.E. and Billingham R.E. (1977)
          Transplantation Proc. 9: 1477.
37.   Lefevre ME.E., Hammer R. and Joel D.D. (1979) J. Reticuloend.
          Soc. 26: 553.
38.   Challacombe S., Krco C.J., David C.S. and Tomasi T.B. (1980)
          (submitted).
39.   Gearhart G.J. and Cebra J.J. (1979) J. Exp. Med. 149: 216.
40.   Macpherson G.G. and Steer H.W. (1979) in "Function and Structure
          of the Immune System", ed. Muller-Bucholtz W. and Muller-
          Hermelink, Plenum Press, New York, p. 433.
41.   Falchuk K.R., Walker W.A., Perrott J.L. and Isselbacher K.J.
          (1977) Infect. Immun. 17: 361.
42.   Svennerholm A-M., Holmgren J., Hanson L.A., Lindblad B.S.
          Quereshi F. and Rahimtoola R-J. (1977) Scand. J. Immunol. 6:
          1345.
43.   Lawrence G., Shann F., Freestone D.S. and Walker P.D. (1979)
          Lancet 1: 227.
44.   Sturn B. and Schneweis K.E. (1978) Med. Microbiol. Immunol.
          165: 119.
45.   Nichols R.L., Murray E.S. and Nisson P.E. (1978) J. Infect. Dis.
          138: 742.
46.   Swarbrick E.T., Stokes C.R. and Soothill J.F. (1979) Gut 20: 121.
47.   Pierce N.F. and Koster F.T. (1980) J. Immunol. 124: 307.
48.   Parker D. and Turk J.L. (1978) Int Arch. Allergy Appl. Immun.
          57: 289.
49.   Asherson G.L., Zembala M., Pereira M.A.C.C., Mayhew B. and
          Thomas W.R. (1977) Cell. Immunol. 33: 145.
50.   Mattingly J.A., Eardley D.D., Kemp J.D. and Gershon R.K. (1979)
          J. Immunol. 122: 787.
51.   Mattingly J.A. and Waksman B.H. (1978) J. Immunol. 121: 1878.
52.   Chalon M.P., Milne R.W. and Vaerman J-P. (1979) Eur. J.
          Immunol. 9: 747.
53.   Nagan J. and Kind L.S. (1978) J. Immunol. 120: 861.
54.   Amsden A., Ewan V., Yoshida T. and Cohen S. (1978) J. Immunol.
          122: 838.
56.   McGhee J.R., Kiyono H., Michalek S.M., Babb J.L., Rosenstrei
          Rosenstreich D.L. and Mergenhagen S.E. (1980) J. Immunol.
          124: 1603.
57.   Pittard, W.B. and Bill K. (1979) Cell. Immunol. 42: 437.

58. Hoerlein A.B. (1957) J. Immunol. 78: 112.
59. Jarrett E.E.E. and Hall E. (1979) Nature 280: 145.

THE HANDLING OF INGESTED ANTIGENS

E.T. Swarbrick

St. Bartholomew's Hospital
London EC1, U.K.

The surface area of the intestine is one factor which makes it such an effective absorptive organ but it also permits considerable exposure to the enormous quantities of antigenic material within its lumen. The intestinal mucosa is widely thought to be impermeable to large molecular weight substances and food is generally absorbed in digested form. However, if the contents of the intestine act as antigens they must cross the external chemical and physical barriers in the lumen and gain access to the immune mechanisms within the body. That macromolecules are absorbed has been suspected since 1864 when Stokvis showed that after the ingestion of large amounts of egg proteins patients developed proteinuria and he suggested that some protein was being absorbed intact and secreted by the kidney.

Absorption of macromolecules by the intestine occurs in all mammals so far tested. There is good evidence that neonatal and young animals absorb more than adults although the evidence in man is indirect and less good. Neonatal ruminants, who derive all their passive immunity after birth, absorb large quantities of intact proteins of all kinds from colostrum and milk in the first two to three days of life[1]. At this time such 'bulk transport' ceases -- a process known as 'closure' -- and little is absorbed subsequently. 'Closure' relates to mucosal maturity and is controlled by unknown colostral factors since early feeding causes premature closure while starvation delays it.

Rodents acquire some of their passive immunity by the specific absorption of intact immunoglobulin (Ig) from milk[2]. This process goes on for 18 days and ceases comparatively abruptly, none being absorbed after 21 days. Antibodies can be detected in the circulation of 12 day old rats within 30 minutes of intragastric administration

and reach a peak in 3 hours. This process is specific for homologous
Ig's and can be blocked by the Fc portion but not the Fab portion of
the Ig[3]; these observations suggest receptor-mediated transport.
Species-specific binding of IgG to isolated brush borders and intra-
cellular cytoplasmic membranes of neonatal, but not adult, rodents,
has been demonstrated[4].

'Closure' in rodents seems to be directly related to the maturity
of enzyme systems and therefore presumably of cell membranes. This
may account for the loss of Ig receptors. It can be accelerated by
steroid administration[5].

There is no evidence of specific Ig absorption or bulk transport
of colostral protein in human babies, and although non-specific
macromolecular absorption may occur to a greater extent in babies
than in adults, the quantities involved are very small and closure
in the true sense of the word does not occur after birth.

Cow's milk antigens are detectable in the serum of most infants
within approximately two weeks of weaning, no matter when it
occurs[6]. The production of antibodies to these proteins starts at
two weeks and is present in almost all by three months. The incidence
of antigenaemia is reduced by this time and is almost nil after one
year, by which time the incidence of circulating antibodies is also
falling so that none of the subjects have any detectable antibodies
by five years. Although this study was only semiquantitative the
high levels of antibodies to food proteins has been confirmed in
infants[7] and since less antigen or antibody was detected in older
children or adults it may be concluded that less antigen is absorbed.
An alternative possibility is that the circulating antibodies were
effectively eliminating the antigen. It is interesting to note that
it has been proposed that specific immune mechanisms might exclude
antigens[6]. Macromolecular absorption has been shown to be energy
dependant in that it can be reduced by inhibitors of oxidative
phosphorylation and glycolysis[8].

Electron microscopic studies of both immunoglobulins[9] and
heterologous proteins[8] suggest that intact protein molecules
aggregate on the enterocyte surface and are taken into the cells by
pinocytosis. The pinocytotic vacuoles traverse the cell and coalesce
with lysosomes to form phagolysosomes. Some, perhaps the majority
of protein is digested but some remains undigested and is discharged
into the lateral spaces. The receptor specific binding of Ig may
protect it from lysosomal digestion permitting most to reach the
circulation intact[10]. There is no satisfactory evidence to support
the absorption of macromoleucles between the cells across tight
junctions.

Hypotheses based on electron microscopy may be criticised on the grounds that the appearances may be artefactual[11] but several systems of receptor-mediated endocytosis, in addition to Ig absorption, by neonatal animals are known to exist[12] and the rapid entry of, for example, radiolabelled low-density lipoproteins visualised by electron microscopy precisely parallels the biochemically derived data on their uptake and degradation. Such results vindicate the use of electron microscopy to some extent. Receptor-binding and the migration of receptor-bound molecules to 'coated pits' leads to rapid internalisation but the mechanisms for initiating non receptor-mediated pinocytosis are unknown.

The fate of intact macromolecules once they have traversed the epithelial cell is not fully elucidated but between one third and one half of that which is absorbed enters the circulation via the lymphatics and the remainder via the portal blood[13,14]. Little is known about such partitioning in man but endotoxins have been found in the protal blood of normals when it is absent from the systemic circulation[15]. The actual amounts absorbed are difficult to calculate since the usual methods of study involving the rate of disappearance from the lumen are invalidated by intraluminal digestion. Whole body studies in rats of protein-bound radio-activity[16] and calculations based on partitioning[13,14] suggest that for heterologous proteins it is between 0.2% and 2% of the total administered.

The factors controlling the absorption of antigen may be both non-specific and specific. Gastric acid and pancreatic and mucosal enzymes will denature and digest proteins and reduce their availability. Evidence to support this comes from the observations that oral immunisation is more effective when antigens are administered with bicarbonate[17,18,19] and that following the ligation of the pancreatic duct the absorption of insulin is enhanced[20]. The maturity and integrity of these systems may alter significantly the handling of ingested antigens in disease.

Many early workers believed that protein passed unchanged through the mucosa only if bile or other irritants damaged the mucosa and made it more permeable[21,22]. Others observed that children suffering from gastrointestinal disturbances can be sensitised to foods which they tolerated prior to their illness[23]. Food antigens were found in the blood of malnourished children[24,25] and those recovering from gastroenteritis[26]. The presence of increased antifood antibodies in coeliac disease[27,28], ulcerative colitis[29] and malnutrition[30] has been interpreted as showing increased leakiness.

In other phagocytotic systems the amount of substrate absorbed depends upon its adsorption to the cell surface which depends upon the net charge. In an everted gut sac experimental alteration of the surface charge results in altered absorption into the sac[31]. Diseases could alter the mucosal surface charge.

Antigen specific mechanisms of immune exclusion were first hinted at by Lippard et al[6] and were predicted by Heremans[32] who suggested that the 'antifouling' paint of secretory IgA would reduce antigen absorption. In rats the prior feeding of bovine serum albumin (BSA) or horseradish peroxidase (HRP) reduced their subsequent absorption[33].

Four groups including our own have now reported immune exclusion in vivo[34,35,36,37]. In our experiments mice were fed 25 mg ovalbumin daily for fourteen days; fourteen days later levels of ovalbumin in their blood were reduced after the administration of 40 mg intragastrically as measured by radio-immuno-assay. The feeding of antigen might induce circulating antibodies which could eliminate any absorbed antigen from the circulation. Other groups have not considered this possibility but we tested it by administering intra-venously radio-labelled ovalbumin to similarly treated groups of mice. The decline in intravenous radio-activity was the same for mice previously fed ovalbumin as for controls given saline. The differences in serum concentration between experimental and control animals after ingestion are therefore not due to differences of immune elimination but may be due to differences in absorption.

The mechanism of such antigen exclusion has been elucidated to some extent and seems to be a function of local immunoglobulin. In a series of in vitro experiments using everted gut sacs there is increased initial adsorption of labelled antigen on to the mucosa of parenterally immunised animals[38] and the antigen removed from the surface by gentle washing is in the form of an immune complex coupled to IgGa. There is also increased digestion of labelled antigen after prolonged incubation in the presence of immune gut sacs[38] but this is reduced if the pancreatic duct has previously been ligated[39]. Preformed antibody-antigen complexes in two-fold antibody excess stimulate goblet cell disruption and mucus secretion secretion[36] as does the administration of intestinal antigen to orally immunised animals[19].

A unifying hypothesis has been proposed that mucosal antibody binds free immunal antigens stimulating mucus secretion[40] which then prevents antigenic contact with the epithelial cell by enhancing its mechanical removal and thus reducing its absorption. In addition the intraluminal digestion of antigenic protein by pancreatic proteases is increased by its binding to specific antibody.

It has been proposed that immune exclusion is a function of the "antifouling paint" of sIgA[32] which is an elegant suggestion because sIgA is intimately bound to the mucus, possibly by sulphydryl binding to cystine residues, and secretor piece apparently protects it from proteolytic digestion[41,42]. The MOPC 315 myeloma IgA with antibody-like affinity for Dnp reduces the absorption of Dnp-linked proteins in the bronchial tree of rats[43] but it has not been possible to show immune exclusion directly in mice with myeloma as the circulating IgA will eliminate any absorbed antigen from the circulation[44]. The immune exclusion of HSA by rats with mucosal scrapings containing IgA antibodies has been passively transferred[34] but others have been unable to demonstrate either circulating or mucosal IgA antibodies after oral immunisation[33]. It remains to be shown that sIgA is responsible for or is capable of immune exclusion.

It is clear that antigen absorption is reduced rather than abolished and BSA can be detected in the serum of normal adults after drinking milk[45]. Most children and some normal adults have circulating antibodies to food proteins which do not appear to do any harm and which presumably are responsible for clearing from the circulation antigens which are absorbed. These antibody responses might be inappropriate in quantity or quality and therefore potentially damaging, but mechanisms exist to ensure this is not the case, namely the induction by feeding of specific immunological tolerance. This is defined as "the specific reduction in response to an antigen induced by prior exposure to the same antigen". It is not a single entity and recent reviews[46,47] have stressed the diversity of possible mechanisms which may be involved.

After feeding egg albumin, oats[48], or zein[49], the usual anaphylactic sensitivity could not be conferred by subsequent injections of the same protein. It was later shown that after feeding dinitrochlorobenzene to rabbits it was impossible to induce skin hypersensitivity to the same substance[50]. More recently it has been shown that feeding HSA to rats, or sheep red blood cells or ovalbumin to mice, reduces the subsequent antibody response to the same antigens when given parenterally[51,52,53,37] and in certain strains of mice the degree of tolerance induced by feeding is greater than by any other means[54].

In parallel experiments to those described above our group has demonstrated that feeding ovalbumin induces both antigen exclusion and specific tolerance simultaneously[37], showing that at least two mechanisms exist to minimise potentially harmful immune responses to otherwise harmless food proteins. Recently it has been shown that Peyer's patch T cells can suppress IgM and IgG synthesis[55] at the same time as stimulating IgA synthesis so mechanisms do exist to explain the paradox.

The relevance to health and disease of these phenomena and their complicated genetic and environmental interactions is unclear but they are likely to be important. The fact that most people are not allergic to ingested antigens must to some extent depend on them, but whether antigen exclusion is more important than tolerance induction or vice versa, or whether both phenomena contribute, needs clarification.

In atopic individuals the clinical response is often dose dependent and allergy has been thought of as "overstimulation" of the IgE mechanisms by excessive amounts of antigen. One possible explanation of the association of atopic allergy with immuno-deficiency particularly for IgA, is a failure of immune exclusion by mucosal antibodies. The concept is supported by the observations that transient IgA deficiency at three months of age predisposes to atopy in children of atopic parents[56] and that exclusive breast feeding reduces the incidence of atopy[57,58]. Furthermore, good evidence for a dose-dependent threshold effect for inducing damaging immune responses to some antigens met naturally, is provided by the observation that over half of all workers in castor oil bean crushing plants will develop atopic symptoms[59]. The dose of antigen administered may therefore be one factor contributing to the induction of allergy or the production of symptoms exclusion is likely to contribute to keeping the dose below the dangerous threshold in otherwise vulnerable individuals.

In order to induce and possibly maintain systemic tolerance, antigen must be absorbed and because the strain of rats which produce large IgE responses to ingested antigens do so with small rather than large antigen doses, it has been suggested that antigen absorption actually helps tolerance induction and presumably exclusion would hinder it[60].

Elson's observations on the role of Peyer's patches in the regulation of local and systemic responses to ingested antigens offer an alternative explanation of the association of IgA deficiency with a number of immunologically mediated conditions including atopic allergy[55]. While transient IgA deficiency in infancy may contribute to the development of atopy by failing to exclude antigen[56] it may simply reflect immaturity of the Peyer's patches associated with failure of tolerance induction, and hence increased susceptibility to mount an atopic response.

IgE mediated responses are often stimulated when the antigen is administered orally and adjuvant is given parenterally[61]. E. coli endotoxin lipopolysaccharide (LPS) might be such an adjuvant and it is present in the intestinal lumen. It can be found in normal portal blood[15] which suggests that it crosses the mucosa and it is possible that such adjuvant action will induce an IgE mediated response in vulnerable individuals.

Bottle-fed infants have a predominantly coliform flora; perhaps breast feeding reduces the incidence of atopic allergy not only by reducing antigenic load but also by reducing the adjuvant action of any antigen that is present during the vulnerable first few months of life.

Circulating antibodies to food proteins are usually taken to reflect antigen absorption and in certain diseases such as ulcerative colitis, Crohn's disease and coeliac disease increased titres suggest increased absorption due to leakiness. Since such antibodies are not known to be damaging the response may be an appropriate physiological way of eliminating circulating antigens harmlessly. The regulatory effects of orally induced tolerance may also be affected in these diseases and such changes may contribute to the high anti-food titres.

Antibodies to cow's milk proteins occur in 80% of children but increasingly fewer adults[62]; but why children have higher titres to milk proteins than adults is not entirely explained. It may result from children drinking more milk than adults but while those adults in Korenblat's study who already had circulating anti-milk antibodies developed a higher titre when immunised orally, those who had no antibody initially developed none suggesting that antigen dose is not the only factor. Those who had no antibodies to start with failed to respond after intradermal immunisation but intradermal immunisation is not, as had been suggested, the same as bypassing the gut since it takes no account of the antigenic form after ingestion, possible adjuvant action, the partitioning of the antigen into vascular and lymphatic compartments nor the function of mucosal lymphoid tissues. Whether the decrease in titre with age is the result of the induction of slow tolerance is not clear but such a phenomenon could explain why children "grow out" of some atopic conditions.

Patients with coeliac disease[63], dermatitis herpetiformis[64] and inflammatory bowel diseases[65] have high levels of circulating immune-complexes but the antigenic component of these complexes is unknown. They may contribute to the extra-intestinal manifestations of inflammatory bowel disease but there is no real evidence that they are damaging. Circulating IgG immune complexes containing milk proteins can be found transiently in normals after drinking milk[44] and may reflect the normal elimination of absorbed antigen.

The relevance of antigen exclusion to the pathogenesis of allergy is perhaps more immediately obvious than to coeliac disease or inflammatory bowel diseases. However, the rare association of IgA deficiency with coeliac disease for example[66] could be related to excessive absorption of the damaging substance or alternatively part of a syndrome in which poor induction of tolerance plays a part[27].

Similar considerations apply in inflammatory bowel diseases[29].
For example it has been suggested that ulcerative colitis is the
result of an immune response to the normal flora. Damaging immune
reactions to the normal flora may be prevented by keeping the appropriate antigen out or by inducing tolerance to it; failure of the
induction of such tolerance or its breakdown might lead to disease.

In order to obtain a better understanding of these diseases
more information is needed about the handling of luminal antigens
both in animals and man. Experiments on tolerance in man are
ethically difficult but studies can be performed on antigen absorption. How much is absorbed? Is there genetically controlled
individual variation? Do neonates absorb more than older children
or adults? Is more absorbed secondary to intestinal disease? How
is the absorbed antigen distributed and what is the role of the
liver? The importance of the way in which the intestine handles
antigens is however obvious, and the work described in animals has
demonstrated the complicated interactions that exist between the
various mechanisms involved.

REFERENCES

1. Morris I.G. (1968) in "Handbook of Physiology" vol. 2 p. 1491,
       Ed. Code C.F., Amer. Physiol. Soc.
2. Halliday R. (1955) Proc. R. Soc. Series B. Biol. Sci 143: 408.
3. Morris I.G. (1963) Proc. R. Soc. London Series B. 157: 160.
4. Jones E.A. and Waldman T. (1972) J. Clin. Invest. 51: 2915.
5. Halliday R. (1959) J. Endocrinol. 18: 56.
6. Lippard V.W., Schloss O.M. and Johnson P.A. (1936) Am. J. Dis.
       Child. 5: 562.
7. Rothberg M. (1969) J. Paediat. 75: 391.
8. Walker W.A., Cornell R., Davenport L.M. and Isselbacher K.J.
       (1972) J. Cell Biol. 54: 195.
9. Clark S.L. (1959) Biophys. Biochem. Cytol. 5: 41.
10. Brambell F.W.R. (1966) Lancet 2: 1087.
11. Hillman H. and Sartory P. (1977) Perception 6: 667.
12. Goldstein J.L., Anderson R.G.W. and Brown M.S. (1979) Nature
       279: 679.
13. Katayama K. and Fujita T. (1972) Biochem. Biophys. Acta 288:
       181.
14. Warshaw A.L., Walker A.W. and Isselbacher K.J. (1974) Gastro-
       enterology 66 987.
15. Jacob A.I., Goldberg P.K., Bloom N., Degenshein M.D. and
       Kozinn P.J. (1977) Gastroenterology 72: 1268.
16. Hemmings W.A. and Williams E.W. (1978) Gut 19: 715.
17. Northrup R.S., Bienenstock J. and Tomasi T.B. (1970) J. Infect.
       Dis. 121: 137.
18. Dupont H.L., Formal S.B. and Hornick R.S. (1971) N. Eng. J. Med.
       285: 1.

19. Lake A.M., Bloch K.J., Neutra M.R. and Walker W.A. (1979)
        J. Immunol. 122: 834.
20. Danforth E. and Moore R.O. (1959) Endocrinology 5: 118.
21. Arloing F. and Langeran L. (1923) Compte. Rend. Soc. de Biol.
        89: 1293 cited by Ratner & Gruehl (1934).
22. Makaroff (1923) Compte. Rend. Soc. de Biol. 89: 286 cited by
        Ratner & Gruehl (1934).
23. Hutinel (1908) Clinique, Paris, 3: 227 cited by Ratner & Gruehl
        (1934).
24. Schloss O.M. and Worthen T.W. (1916) Am. J. Dis. Child. II: 342.
25. Anderson A.F. and Schloss O.M. (1923) Am. J. Dis. Child. 26:
        451.
26. Gruskay F.L. and Cooke R.E. (1955) Paediatrics 16: 763.
27. Taylor K.B., Turelove S.C., Thomson D.L. and Wright R. (1961)
        BMJ ii: 1727-1731.
28. Kumar P.J., Ferguson A., Lancaster-Smith M. and Clark M.L. (1976)
        Scan. J. Gastroent. 11: 5.
29. Taylor K.B. and Truelove S.C. (1973) Lancet ii: 924.
30. Chandra R.K. (1975) Arch. Dis. Child. 50: 532.
31. Smith M.W. and Burton K.E. (1972) Anim. Prod. 15: 139.
32. Heremans J.F. (1969) "The Secretory Immunologic System" p. 309,
        Nat. Inst. Child Health and Human Dev., Bethesda.
33. Walker W.A., Isselbacher K.J. and Bloch K.J. (1972) Science
        177: 608
34. Andre C., Lambert R., Bazin H. and Heremans J.F. (1974) Eur. J.
        Immunol. 4: 701.
35. Seifert J., Ring J., Steininger J. and Brendel W. (1977) Nutr.
        Metab. 21 (suppl. I): 256.
36. Walker W.A., and Bloch K.J. (1977) Gastroenterology (Abstract)
        A162/1185.
37. Swarbrick E.T., Stokes C.R. and Soothill J.F. (1979) Gut 20:
        121-125.
38. Walker W.A., Wu M., Isselbacher K.J. and Bloch K.J. (1975)
        J. Immunol. 115: 854.
39. Walker W.A., Wu M., Isselbacher K.J. and Bloch K.J. (1975)
        Gastroenterology 69: 1223.
40. Walker W.A., Wu M. and Bloch K.J. (1977) Science 197: 370.
41. Brown W.R., Newcomb R.W. and Ishizaka K. (1970) J. Clin. Invest.
        49: 1374.
42. Steward M.W. (1971) Biochem. Biophys. Acta 236: 440.
43. Stokes C.R., Soothill J.F. and Turner M.W. (1975) Nature 255:
        745.
44. Swarbrick E.T., Stokes C.R. and Soothill J.F. (1976) Gut 18:
        A945.
45. Paganelli R., Levinsky R.J., Brostoff J. and Wraith D.G. (1979)
        Lancet i: 1270.
46. British Medical Bulletin (May 1976) 32 (2).
47. Waksman B.H. (1977) Clin. Exp. Immunol. 28: 363-374.
48. Wells H.G. (1911) J. Infect. Dis. 9: 147.
49. Wells H.G. and Osborne T.B. (1911) J. Infect. Dis. 8: 66.

50. Chase M.W. (1946) Proc. Soc. Bio. (N.Y.) 61: 257.
51. Thomas H.C. and Parrott D.M.V. (1974) Immunology 27: 631-639.
52. Andre C., Heremans J.F., Vaerman J.P. and Cambiaso C.L. (1975)
         J. Exp. Med. 142: 1509.
53. Hanson D.G., Vaz N.M., Maa L.C.S., Hornbrook M.M., Lynch J.M.
         and Roy C.A. (1977) Int. Archs. Allergy Appl. Immun. 55: 526.
54. Vaz N.M., Maia L.C.S., Hanson D.G. and Lynch J.M. (1977) J.
         Allergy Clin. Immunol. 60: 110-115.
55. Elson C.O., Heck J.A. and Strober W.E. (1979) J. Exp. Med. 149:
         632.
56. Taylor B., NOrman A.P., Orgel H.A., Stokes C.R., Turner M.W.
         and Soothill J.F. (1973) Lancet ii: 111-113.
57. Matthew D.J., Taylor B., Norman A.P., Turner M.W. and
         Soothill J.F. (1977) Lancet i: 321.
58. Saarinen N.M., Kajasuari M., Backman A. and Siimes M. (1979)
         Lancet ii: 163.
59. Ordmann D. (1955) Int. Archs. Allergy. App. Immunol. 7: 10.
60. Jarrett E.E.E. (1977) Lancet II 223.
61. Bazin H. and Platteau B. (1976) Immunol. 30: 679.
62. Rothberg R.M. and Farr R.S. (1965) Paediatrics 35: 571.
63. Doe W.F., Booth C.C. and Brown D.L. (1973) Lancet i: 402.
64. Mowbray J.F., Holborrow E.J., Hoffbrand A.V., Seah P.P. and
         Fry L. (1973) Lancet i: 400.
65. Jewell D.P. and Maclennan I.C.M. (1973) Clin. Exp. Immunol.
         14: 219.
66. Asquith P., Thompson R.A. and Cooke W.T. (1969) Lancet ii: 129.

HANDLING OF FOOD ANTIGENS AND THEIR COMPLEXES BY

NORMAL AND ALLERGIC INDIVIDUALS

R.J. Levinsky, R. Paganelli, D.M. Robertson,
and D.J. Atherton

Department of Immunology
Institute of Child Health
30 Guilford Street
London WC1, U.K.

The gastrointestinal tract, in addition to its main function as a digestive organ which absorbs nutrients, provides a barrier against the entry of macromolecular antigen. This barrier is incomplete for there is now ample evidence that antigen crosses the gastrointestinal mucosa in all healthy individuals[1]. The amounts which enter the circulation are insignificant nutritionally but are sufficient to immunise since antibodies to food proteins may be demonstrated to low titres in most healthy people[2]. These antibodies are apparently not damaging and hypersensitivity reactions to food proteins are uncommon.

Oral immunisation elicits a local immune response in which secretory IgA antibody (SIgA) complexes with antigen within the gut lumen thereby substantially reducing antigen entry into the circulation[3]. In addition to this local immune mechanism, a state of systemic hyporesponsiveness or "oral tolerance" is produced in which the individual is incapable of mounting an appropriate antibody response when the same antigen is subsequently given parenterally[4,5,6]. The mechanisms for maintaining this state of oral tolerance are not understood but there is evidence from studies in mice that serum factors such as immune complexes[7], or IgG_1 antibody[8] may be involved. Suppressor T cells may be generated by oral antigen administration, but as this is only transient it is unlikely to provide the entire answer[9].

Food allergy may be regarded as a major breakdown in oral tolerance. In order to understand some of the mechanisms involved in food tolerance and how this breakdown results in damage to food

allergic patients, we have studied food antigen handling by the gut
in healthy individuals and compared their responses to those obtained
in food allergic patients.

ANTIGEN ENTRY IN THE NEWBORN INFANT

     In many species of animals, a great deal of the passive acqui-
sition of maternal immunoglobulin is derived via breast feeding.
The gut is initially freely permeable to macromolecules and after a
variable time in different species abruptly closes to form tight
junctions. This phenomenon, known as gut closure, may be enhanced
by certain factors in colostrum[10]. Food antigen entry has been
reported in normal healthy babies as early as five days after
birth[11], but in no greater amounts than that absorbed by older
children. In order to see if gut closure occurs in man, we have
studied food antigen entry in premature babies. The babies'
gestational age ranged from 28 to 40 weeks and each baby was studied
24 hours after the introduction of a cow's milk based formula (SMA)
given hourly by nasogastric tube. The amounts fed were related to
birthweight. A blood sample was taken 30 minutes after the feed.
Several of the babies were initially started on breast milk but
because the milk flow was inadequate the feeds were changed to the
SMA formula after the first 24 hours. These babies were also given
the formula feed before study. Using a solid phase radioimmunoassay
to measure serum levels of β lactoglobulin[12], a protein which is
present to a concentration of 3 mg/ml in cows' milk, we have shown
that many of the very premature infants absorb considerably greater
quantities of antigenically intact protein than do full term babies.

     There was great variation in the levels of β lactoglobulin
absorbed but several of the very premature babies absorbed as much
as 70-80 ng/ml, an enormous amount in comparison to that absorbed
by healthy adults (see later). Only two premature infants in the
older gestational age group absorbed moderately large amounts.
These findings suggest that gut closure is a pre-term event in humans
and, although there is great variation, has occurred usually by the
36th week of gestation.

Table 1.   Levels of β lactoglobulin in premature infants.

Gestational Age	28-35 weeks	35-40 weeks
1. SMA only	(n-12) mean 9.7 ng/ml (range 0.1-100 ng/ml)	(n=6) mean 5.0 ng/ml (range 0-25 ng/ml)
2. Breast milk for 24 hours then SMA	(n=5) mean 4.9 ng/ml (range 0-24 ng/ml)	NONE

It is interesting that those very premature infants who initially were fed breast milk before going on to the cows' milk based formula did not absorb such large amounts, indicating that some factor in breast milk enhanced gut closure in these infants.

ANTIGEN ABSORPTION IN HEALTHY ADULTS

Five healthy non-atopic adults were studied by taking sequential blood samples over a five hour period following the ingestion of 1.2 litres of fresh cows' milk. The blood samples were analysed for free circulating β lactoglobulin[12], for immune complexes containing IgG and for IgA[13], for Clq binding immune complexes[14] and for the antigen within the immune complexes[15]. This latter technique involves immune complex enrichment by polyethylene glycol precipitation; the complex is then dissociated in acid buffer and the constituents are adsorbed on to a plastic surface. After neutral pH washing, the antigen is detected by using a radiolabelled antigen. Radioactive counts bound to the plastic solid phase give an indication of either antigen or antibody concentration within the immune complex.

After drinking 1.2 litres of milk, β lactoglobulin was found in the circulation within 30 minutes; in most of the individuals a second peak of absorption was demonstrated at 4-5 hours. The levels attained in all subjects were no greater than 3 ng/ml. This two peak distribution of antigen was a consistent finding and since it also occurs in animals never previously exposed to the antigen, it probably represents two different routes of absorption, the first into the portal circulation and the slower one into the lymphatics and then into the circulation.

We have previously demonstrated circulating soluble immune complexes following milk ingestion in healthy subjects[15]. When these sera were analysed for the type of immune complex there was very little variation in the levels of IgG and Clq binding immune complexes, but all the subjects studied showed a large rise in IgA complexes again occurring within 30 minutes of ingestion and falling to baseline after approximately 90 minutes. Using the immune complex splitting technique, both β lactoglobulin and bovine serum albumin (BSA) have been demonstrated to be antigenic constituents of these complexes. A representative profile of β lactoglobulin absorption, IgA, IgG and Clq binding complexes and the two antigens within the complexes is shown in Fig. 1.

These results indicate that serum IgA is involved in clearing antigens from the circulation; the fact that monomeric IgA does not activate complement or elicit other damaging reactions makes it the ideal class of immunoglobulin for safely eliminating circulating food proteins. It is possible that the small amounts of antigen continually entering the circulation via the gastrointestinal mucosa is a necessary prerequisite for maintaining an effective IgA antibody

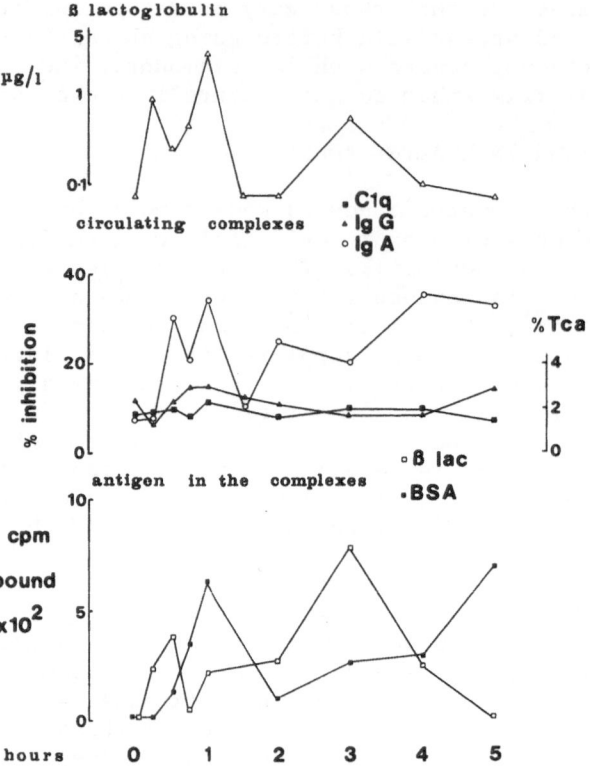

Fig. 1.   Representative profile of antigen absorption
          (β lactoglobulin) and immune complex formation (IgG, IgA
          and Clq binding complexes) in a healthy non-atopic adult
          after drinking 1.2 litres of fresh cows' milk. Both
          bovine serum albunim and β lactoglobulin were shown to be
          antigenic constituents of the IgA immune complexes.

response. T lymphocytes have been demonstrated in Peyer's patches
which enhance IgA production while suppressing IgM and IgG[16].
The route of antigen entry must be equally important for Peyer's
patch lymphocytes respond to enteric, but not parenteral antigens
with preferential IgA class antibodies[17]. We have recently
demonstrated that the same is true for human tonsillar cells which
produced specific IgA antibody predominantly when stimulated with
β lactoglobulin but specific IgM and IgG antibodies when stimulated
in tissue culture with tetanus toxoid (Paganelli and Levinsky,
unpublished).

      Hence it is likely that the route of antigen entry as well as
the unique microenvironment of the gut-associated lymphoid system
is important for maintaining the IgA immune response both at local

and systemic levels and thereby providing a safe mechanism for
dealing with enteric antigens. These observations do not explain
the mechanisms of oral food tolerance; we still do not know how
circulating IgA immune complexes are handled by the reticuloendothelial system or whether any serum factor acts as a negative feedback to maintain systemic hyporesponsiveness. In mice, IgG_1 antibody
provides such feedback control[8], but this is not necessarily true
for man and we must retain an open mind as to whether serum IgA in
complexed form plays any part in oral food tolerance.

ANTIGEN ENTRY IN FOOD ALLERGIC SUBJECTS

     The symptoms of food allergy are numerous; it may produce local
gut effects such as the bleeding and diarrhoea of cows' milk
allergy[18], systemic effects such as skin rashes, urticaria or
eczema[19], asthma[20], migrane[21] and there are even reports of
patients with rheumatoid arthritis in whom joint symptoms are substantially improved by a diet free of certain foods[22].

     We have studied food antigen entry in children and adults with
food allergy in whom the predominant symptoms were eczema, but some
of the patients experienced bronchospasm after ingestion of either
milk or eggs. The patients were given a cocktail of raw eggs and
milk to drink; the amount administered was according to body weight.
All of the patients were skin-prick tested to individual milk and
egg antigens and a dietary history of symptom exacerbation in
response to either foodstuff obtained. Using the same techniques,
we estimated free circulating antigen (β lactoglobulin and ovalbumin),
IgG, IgA and C1q binding immune complexes and the antigens contained
within the immune complexes. Higher levels of free circulating
antigen (up to 15 ng/ml) were obtained in the food allergic patients
than in the healthy non-atopic subjects who were fed an equivalent
antigenic load. In contrast to the IgA immune complexes formed in
response to food challenge in the non-atopic individuals, the food
allergic individuals formed immune complexes containing IgG and
IgE[23] as well as C1q binding ones[15]. These immune complexes were
shown to contain the food antigens β lactoglobulin and ovalbumin by
means of the immune complex splitting technique. In the majority
of the patients the two peak distribution of antigen entry and
immune complex formation was observed. Of interest was the
observation that those patients who were skin-prick test positive
to the ingested food produced predominantly IgG and C1q binding
complexes, whereas the skin test negative patients had higher levels
of IgA complexes.

     The drug sodium cromoglycate is thought to prevent mast cell
degranulation by inhibiting the calcium influx across the cell
membrane. When patients were pretreated with 1 gm of oral sodium
cromoglycate prior to ingestion of the milk/egg cocktail, not only
were the symptoms of skin itching and wheezing abolished, but antigen
entry and immune complex formation were substantially reduced (Fig. 2).

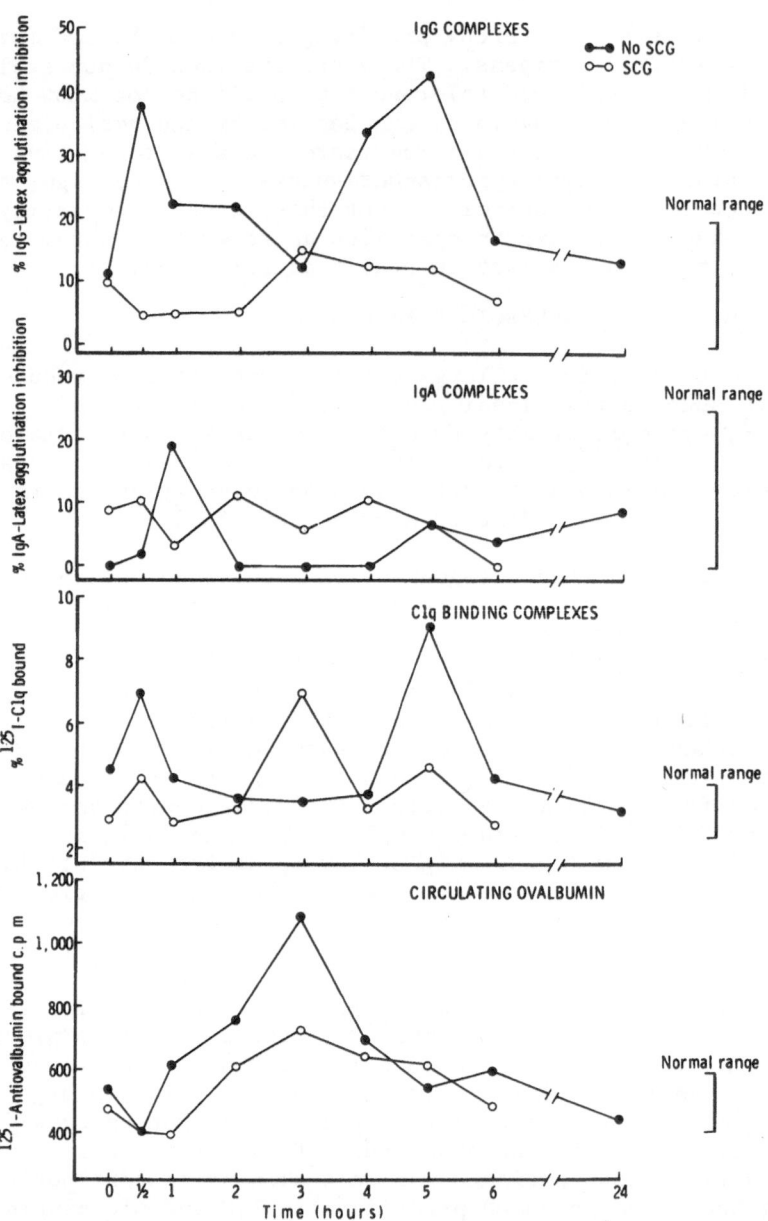

Fig. 2. Representative profile of antigen absorption (ovalbumin) and
         immune complex formation in a food allergic patient with
         eczema and asthma. The complexes following ingestion of two
         lightly boiled eggs contained ovalbumin and were pre-
         dominantly IgG and C1q binding. Prior treatment with oral
         sodium cromoglycate blocked much of the antigen entry and
         immune complex formation as well as abolishing symptoms of
         bronchospasm. (Reproduced with permission, Lancet (1979)
         i: 1270.)

PATHOGENESIS OF ATOPIC ECZEMA

It is important to note the differences in the types of immune response obtained after food ingestion. Normal subjects produced IgA immune complexes predominantly, but in the food allergic subjects the major responses were ones of IgG, Clq binding and IgE immune complexes.

In the food allergic subject the central role of local production of specific IgE in the intestinal mucosa can be envisaged. Even low levels of sensitisation can cause mast cell degranulation upon allergen challenge; the increased vascular permeability allows further antigen entry with subsequent immune complex formation. Any of the immunoglobulin classes may be involved in immune complex formation, but those that cause complement activation (IgM and IgG) provoke most damage. Localisation of immune complexes within an organ is facilitated by local increase in vascular permeability[24]. Complement fixing antigen excess immune complexes may localise in skin or lungs by triggering antigen specific IgE sensitised mast cells to release histamine, platelet activating factor and other mediators of vascular permeability. With complement activation, chemotactic factors are released to attract neutrophils and mononuclear phagocytes which accentuate the inflammatory response by release of proteolytic enzymes.

This hypothetical injury mechanism does not fully account for the small round cell infiltration which occurs in the skin of patients with atopic eczema[25], but histamine may also be chemotactic for lymphocytes, thus amplifying this mechanism[26]. Similar lesions may also be produced experimentally when immune complexes in suitable proportions are injected into the skin of animals[27].

These observations in food allergy provide evidence for the inter-relationships of Type I IgE mediated and Type III immune complex mediated hypersensitivity reactions. They may provide the explanation for the "late" 6 hour responses that have been observed in a variety of clinical situations in association with Type I hypersensitivity reactions[28,29]. Sodium cromoglycate is a poorly absorbed drug and its effect in food allergy is probably by local inhibition of gut mast cell degranulation, thereby reducing vascular permeability and further antigen entry. The fact that both early and late reactions were blocked by this drug further emphasises the close inter-relationship of hypersensitivity injury mechanisms.

ACKNOWLEDGEMENTS

We are grateful to the Nuffield Foundation (R.P.), the M.R.C. (D.J.A.) and Fisons Ltd. (R.J.L.) for financial support.

REFERENCES

1. Walker W.A. and Isselbacher K.J. (1974) Gastroenterology 67:
    531.
2. Peterson R.D.A. and Good R.A. (1965) Pediatrics 31: 209.
3. Ogra P.L. and Karzon D.T. (1970) Paed. Clin. North Amer. 17:
    385.
4. Chase M.S. (1946) Proc. of Soc. Exp. Biol. and Med. (N.Y.) 61:
    257.
5. Thomas H.C. and Parrott D.M.V. (1974) Immunology 27: 631.
6. Swarbrick E.J., Stokes C.R. and Soothill J.F. (1979) Gut 20:
    121.
7. Andre C., Heremans J.F., Vaerman J.P. and Cambiaso (1975)
    J. Exp. Med. 142: 1509.
8. Chalon M.P., Milne R.W. and Vaerman J.P. (1979) Eur. J. of Imm.
    9: 747.
9. Richman L.K., Chiller J.M., Brown W.R., Hanson D.G. and Vaz N.M.
    (1979) J. Immunol. 121: 2429.
10. Walker W.A. (1979) in "Development of Mammalian Absorptive
    Processes", Ciba Foundation Symposium 70: 201.
11. Gruskay F.L. and Cooke R.E. (1955) Pediatrics 16: 763.
12. Paganelli R. and Levinsky R.J. (1980) J. Imm. Methods (in press).
13. Levinsky R.J. and Soothil J.F. (1977) J. Exp. Med. 142: 1509.
14. Zubler R.H., Lange G., Lambert P.H. and Miescher P.A.,
    J. Immunol. 116: 232.
15. Paganelli R., Levinsky R.J., Brostoff J. and Wraith D.G. (1979)
    Lancet i: 1270.
16. Elson C.O., Heck J.A. and Strober W. (1979) J. Exp. Med. 149:
    632.
17. Gearhart P.J. and Cebra J.J. (1979) J. Exp. Med. 149: 216.
18. Collins-Williams C. (1962) Int. Arch. of Allergy 20: 38.
19. Atherton D.J., Soothill J.F., Sewell M., Wells R.S. and
    Chilvers C.E.D. (1978) Lancet 1: 401.
20. Buisseret P.D. (1978) Lancet i: 304.
21. Monro J., Brostoff J., Carini C. and Zilka K. (1980) Lancet ii:
    1.
22. Catterall W.E. (1979) Ann. Rheum. Dis. 36: 594.
23. Brostoff J., Carini C., Wraith D.G., Paganelli R. and
    Levinsky R.J. (1979) in "The Mast Cell" ed. Pepys J. and
    Edwards A.M., Pitman, London, p. 380.
24. Cochrane C.G. and Hawkins D. (1968) J. Exp. Med. 127: 137.
25. Mihm M.C., Soter N.A., Dvorak H. and Austen K.F. (1976) J.
    Invest. Derm. 67: 305.
26. Smorgorzewska E., Layward L. and Soothill J.F. (1980) Clin.
    Exp. Immunol. (in press).
27. Spector W.G. and Heeson W. (1969) J. Path. Bact. 98: 32.
28. Pelikan E. (1978) Ann. Allergy 41: 37.
29. Solley G.O., Gleich G.J., Jordon R.E. and Schrocter A.L. (1976)
    J. Clin. Invest. 58: 408.

BACTERIOSTATIC SYSTEMS IN HUMAN MILK

J.J. Bullen

National Institute for Medical Research
Mill Hill
London NW7 1AA

Before considering the composition of human milk and its protective properties for the infant it is worth emphasising that primates (and guinea-pigs) have the advantage over many other animals in that the transmission of passsive immunity is largely prenatal[1]. This is vital for the prevention of bacterial invasion from the gut. Animals with epitheliochorial placentation like the pig and calf, if deprived of colostrum, almost invariably die of septicaemia since they normally absorb protective IgG from colostrum during the first few hours of life. Human babies deprived of colostrum and milk lack protective factors in the gut and may suffer severe diarrhoea which can sometimes be fatal. Nevertheless their susceptibility to bacterial invasion from the gut is greatly reduced when compared with other milk deprived animals.

ANTIBACTERIAL FACTORS IN HUMAN MILK

Human colostrum contains about 5 mg of secretory IgA per ml and mature milk about 2 mg per ml[2]. Fairly constant levels of IgA (14 mg per g of milk protein) are reached by about 5 days post partum. IgM immunoglobulin is present in colostrum at approximately 29 mg/g milk protein but this declines to about 3-4 mg/g protein by the 120th day. IgG is present in only small amounts (1-5 mg/g milk protein) in both colostrum and milk[3]. As far as antibodies are concerned, high titres have been found against O antigens of E. coli representing the serogroups responsible for 31 out of 43 outbreaks of infection in the newborn[4]. These antibodies are largely of the secretory IgA class[5]. In the newborn infant little digestion of protein takes place in the stomach[6]. The milk IgA is also resistant to digestion in the gut as a whole and can be detected in the faeces[4].

31

Another major component of human milk is the iron-binding protein lactoferrin. In colostrum it is present in concentrations as high as 6 mg/ml but this falls to 2-3 mg/ml after 5 days. Transferrin is also present but only in small amounts (10-50 µg/ml)[7]. Both proteins are only partially saturated with iron[8].

Human milk also contains about 4×10^5 cells per ml of which 20-80% are polymorphs and the rest macrophages, lymphocytes and eosinophils[9]. It also contains large amounts of lysozyme (2-3 mg/ml)[5]. Small amounts of the complement fractions C3 and C4 are also present[10] as well as small amounts of lactoperoxidase[11].

THE PROTECTIVE EFFECT OF HUMAN MILK

There is good evidence that breast feeding protects the human infant against gastroenteritis caused by Escherichia coli. Of the 207 infants with gastroenteritis in Aberdeen in 1947 only four had been entirely breast-fed and in the case of the remaining 203 children, breast feeding had been replaced or supplemented by artificial food for at least a week before the onset of symptoms[12]. In recent years convincing evidence from Guatemala has shown that breast feeding protects agains enteritis caused by E. coli, and against other infections as well. Indeed, breast milk has been used to stop outbreaks of E. coli enteritis when all other forms of treatment, including antibiotics, had failed[13,14].

Pathogenic E. coli causing gastroenteritis must be capable of the following: (1) adherence to the mucosa of the small intestine; (2) production of enterotoxin, and (3) rapid growth in the small intestine[15]. Anti-adhesive effects of antibody have been demonstrated in the pig[16,17,18]. Some of the results obtained with pigs were striking. When piglets from sows which had been vaccinated agains E. coli 0149 were fed 1×10^{10} E. coli 0149 they all survived and there was no evidence that the bacteria adhered to the duodenal mucosa[19]. The duodenal fluid at 3-4 hours after exposure to infection contained about 6×10^7 bacteria per ml whereas the homogenised mucosa, after washing, contained only about 1×10^4 bacteria/ml. In contrast piglets from unvaccinated sows all died and evidence for adhesion of the bacteria to the duodenal mucosa was good since the doudenal contents had about 1×10^9 bacteria per ml and the homogenised mucosa of the washed duodenum about 4×10^8 E. coli per ml. Thus the colostrum from the vaccinated sows reduced adhesion by more than 1000 fold whereas that from non-vaccinated sows had little or no effect.

In babies it is not possible to obtain data similar to that derived from pigs, but there is some evidence that some E. coli strains can adhere to the intestinal mucosa[20] and there is therefore no reason why anti E. coli antibodies in human milk should not have similar anti-adhesive properties. Human IgA may also protect the infant against E. coli enterotoxin[21]. It has been suggested that anti-enterotoxic antibodies are relatively unimportant in pigs[22].

One of the most important protective mechanisms in the small intestine is the suppression of bacterial growth by specific antibody, for which there is ample evidence. The viable counts of entero-pathogenic E. coli in the small intestine of protected pigs may be 1000x to 10,000x less than in unprotected controls[22,23]. In vitro, both human and bovine milk have powerful bacteriostatic effects against pathogenic E. coli[8,18]. Iron binding proteins are essential for this effect. Complement is not required[8,24].

MECHANISM OF INHIBITION OF BACTERIAL GROWTH BY
IRON-BINDING PROTEINS AND ANTIBODY

The iron-binding proteins in milk are normally only partly saturated with iron and have exceptionally high association constants for the metal of about 10^{36}. This means that the amount of free iron in equilibrium with these proteins is only about 10^{-18}M which is far too low for normal bacterial growth. In order to acquire essential iron the bacteria have to produce chelating agents that have approximately the same association constants for iron as the iron-binding proteins. By this means the bacteria can compete for iron.

An important aspect of understanding bacterial adaptation to growth in a low iron environment is the elucidation of the mechanisms which control the production of the iron chelators. E. coli growing in natural secretions or in defined media containing unsaturated iron-binding proteins secrete enterochelin and, in addition, contain altered species of tRNAs. The tRNAs for phenylalanine, tyrosine and tryptophan elute earlier on chromatography than do the same tRNAs from E. coli growing in media where iron is freely available. These altered tRNAs lack the methylthio moiety of the 2-methylthio-N^6-(Δ^2-isopentenyl) adenosine found adjacent to the anticodon of the tRNAs of the iron replete bacteria. It has been suggested that the tRNA changes play an important part in regulating the expression of operons of the aromatic amino acid biosynthetic pathway[25]. Enterochelin is synthesised by way of a branch of this pathway and multiple control by the amino acids and iron is therefore important in maintaining a balanced metabolism during growth under iron restricted conditions. The same iron related tRNA changes are found in E. coli recovered directly from lethal infections[26]. This strengthens the idea that these changes are important for bacterial growth in vivo and provide an insight into some of the subtle changes that may be required for pathogenicity.

Specific antibody can block the working of the bacterial iron-chelating agents, and so inhibit bacterial growth[27]. Bicarbonate is also essential for the bacteriostatic effect because it is required for the binding of iron by the iron-binding protein, otherwise the citrate in milk allows the bacteria to take up iron as an iron-citrate complex[28]. Adequate amounts of bicoarbonate are probably present in the infant's small intestine[29].

In the experiments shown in Fig. 1 three samples of human milk were centrifuged at 56 000 g for 45 minutes to remove the fat. Bicarbonate was added to the supernatant fluid to give a final concentration of 0.6 per cent. Sterilisation was by filtration through a 0.45 µ Millipore filter. The milk was incubated at 37°C and equilibrated with 5 per cent carbon dioxide in air. This gave a pH of approximately 7.5. Under these conditions the inoculation of the milk with 10^2/ml E. coli 0111 gave rise to a short period of bacterial growth followed by bacteriostasis which lasts for at least 8 hours.

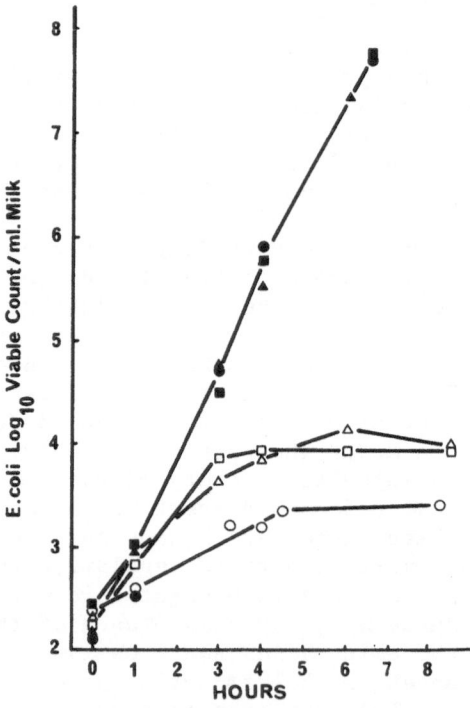

Fig. 1. The bacteriostatic effect of human milk on E. coli 0111 and the effect of adding iron (Δ □ ○ = three samples of human milk; ▲ ■ ● = the same three samples with their iron-binding capacity saturated with iron[8]).

The iron-binding proteins were shown to be essential for bacterial inhibition by the fact that if the unsaturated iron-binding capacity, which varied between 56-89 per cent in the three samples, was saturated with iron by the addition of ferric ammonium citrate then all the bacteriostatic properties of the milk were lost (Fig. 1).

Experiments in tissue culture medium with purified lactoferrin showed that it had only a slight inhibitory effect on E. coli 0111. Antibody alone also had no bacteriostatic effect. However, if a small amount of E. coli antibody was added with lactoferrin then good inhibition was obtained which exactly resembled the effect of milk itself. This showed the importance of the combined effect of antibody and iron-binding protein[8]. Purified IgA has a powerful bacterio-static effect on E. coli, in the presence of lactoferrin, provided the antibody has the correct specificity for the corresponding E. coli serotype[2]. These observations are particularly important since they demonstrate a real antibacterial role for IgA, probably for the first time. Claims[30] that IgA does not enhance the bacteriostatic power of lactoferrin seem unrealistic. Milk from immunoglobulin 'deficient' mothers which had a well-marked bacteriostatic effect on E. coli contained 9 mg IgA/100 ml. This in itself could be sufficient for bacteriostasis and it is scarcely surprising that the addition of more IgA did not enhance this effect.

It has been suggested that porcine milk could have bactericidal effects against E. coli[16,31]. However, all tests made to show this property involved the addition of fresh rabbit serum[31] or fresh pig serum[16] as sources of complement. There is little evi-dence that intestinal fluid contains complement and it has been said that intestinal contents are usually "aggressively anti-complementary"[32]. The invlovement of complement is particularly unlikely in the case of IgA. IgA antibody will not kill Vibrio cholerae in the presence of complement whereas IgM and IgG are highly active[33]. IgA is also a feeble opsonin[33,34]. However, IgA anti-body is highly protective against V. cholerae infection in infant mice[33]. Since the intestinal fluid contains lactoferrin[35,2] it seems highly probable that the IgA operates in concert with this iron-binding protein in the gut.

OTHER POTENTIAL PROTECTIVE SYSTEMS IN MILK

It is difficult to decide whether phagocytic cells in milk provide any protection for the infant. It has been suggested that rat milk leukocytes could protect against enterocolitis in baby rats although there was no definite evidence that protection was due to the bactericidal activity of the cells[36]. Human milk leukocytes can phagocytose bacteria but this is reversed by the addition of ferric ammonium citrate to the whole milk[9], which suggests that the bulk of the antibacterial effect was due to extracellular

lactoferrin and antibody. It is also not known how many leukocytes
would survive in the intestinal tract of babies. Perhaps the phagocytic cells might have real antibacterial function in milk stored
in the mammary gland.

Another factor of unknown value is lysozyme. In porcine milk
there is no relation between the concentration of lysozyme and its
anti E. coli activity. Nor did the removal of lysozyme from milk
by absorption on to bentonite abolish the antibacterial effect[18].
The addition of iron does not have any effect on the titre of haemo-
lytic complement or on the killing of Bacillus megaterium by
lysozyme[37]. Thus the abolition of antibacterial activity by the
addition of iron cannot be attributed ot the inactivation of lysozyme.

It seems unlikely that lactoperoxidase plays any protective
role in human milk. In the first place the concentration of lactoperoxidase in human milk is low, being only about 230 milli units/ml
compared with 22,000 milli units/ml in guinea-pig milk[38]. Secondly
the activity of lactoperoxidase is strongly affected by the pH of the
medium, and is far more effective at pH 5.0 than at pH 7.5[39] and
is not likely to be very effective in the duodenum and small
intestine; in addition anaerobic conditions in the gut could probably
inhibit any antibacterial activity.

EXPERIMENTS WITH ANIMALS

Is there any evidence that the bacteriostatic properties of human
milk against E. coli (Fig. 1) really operate in vivo? It is naturally
impossible to do experiments with babies. Fortunately, guinea-pigs
resemble man to some extent in respect of their placentation[1] and
the composition of their milk. Guinea-pig milk contains lactoferrin
(0.2 to 2 mg/ml) and transferrin (0.2 to 2.0 mg/ml)[7]. When suckling
guinea-pigs were dosed orally with 1×10^6 E. coli 0111 there was a
rapid fall in the viable count of these bacteria, both in the small
and large intestines. After 3 days, counts in the small intestine
were about 10^3/g and in the large intestine about 10^5/g. By this
time the E. coli were greatly outnumbered by a naturally occurring
lactobacillary flora with counts reaching about 10^6/g in the small
intestine and 10^7/g in the large intestine. In contrast to this if
the baby guinea-pigs were fed an artificial milk diet, the numbers
of E. coli 0111 in the small intestine reached 10^9/g, and in the
large intestine 10^{10}/g. It also took much longer for the lactobacillary flora to appear and these bacteria failed to predominate
in either the small or large intestine[8]. This resembles the effect
of feeding babies on artificial diets based on cows' milk[40].

The importance of the iron-binding proteins in guinea-pig milk
was shown by experiments with suckling animals. Newly born guinea-
pigs were divided into two groups. One group was suckled normally
and acted as controls. The other group was also suckled but was

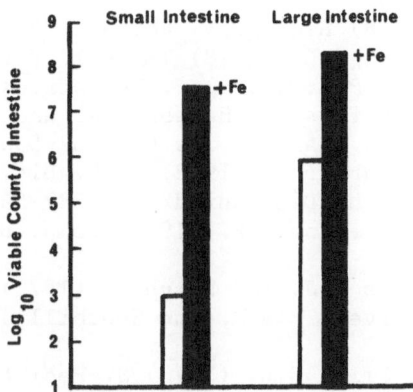

Fig. 2.   The effect of haematin hydrochloride in intestinal
infection with E. coli in suckled guinea-pigs.   (□ = E. coli
in controls; ■ = E. coli in animals fed haematin
hydrochloride[8].

dosed orally with 50 mg of haematin hydrochloride twice daily for
2 days. Both groups received 1×10^6 E. coli 0111 at birth and after
three days counts were made from the small and large intestines. As
anticipated, the controls showed low levels of E. coli in the small
intestine but there was a 100,000 fold increase in numbers of these
bacteria in the animals given haematin hydrochloride (Fig. 2). There
was also a 100 fold increase in the large intestine[8]. This experiment clearly showed the importance of the iron-binding protein in
controlling the growth of E. coli in the gut. Both lactoferrin and
transferrin can only bind ferric iron and haematin hydrochloride
provides a ready source of iron for E. coli. Haematin hydrochloride
has been shown to reverse the bacteriostatic effect of serum and milk
in vitro[24]. The fact that this also happens in vivo strongly
suggests that guinea-pig milk normally has a suppressive effect on
E. coli in the gut, and especially so in the small intestine. There
is every reason to suppose that human milk has the same effect in
babies[8,41] and that this protection in the small intestine is
largely due to the combined effect of IgA antibodies, lactoferrin,
and bicarbonate.

ACKNOWLEDGEMENT

     Figs. 1 and 2 reproduced from Bullen J.J., Rogers H.J. and
Leigh L. (1972) British Medical Journal 1: 69-75, by kind permission
of the Editor.

REFERENCES

1. Brambell F.W. (1958) Biological Reviews 33: 488-531.
2. Rogers H.J. and Synge C. (1978) Immunol. 34: 19-28.
3. Ogra S.S. and Ogra P.L. (1978) J. Pediatrics 92: 546-549.
4. Gindrat J.J., Gothefors L., Hanson L.A. and Winberg J. (1972)
    Acta Paediatrica Scandinavica 61: 587-590.
5. Hanson L.A. and Winberg J. (1972) Arch. Dis. Child. 47: 845-848.
6. Mason S. (1962) Arch. Dis. Child. 37: 387-391.
7. Masson P.L. and Heremans J.F. (1971) Comp. Biochem. and Physiol.
    39B: 119-129.
8. Bullen J.J., Rogers H.J. and Leigh L. (1972) BMJ 1: 69-75.
9. Robinson J.E., Harvery B.A.M. and Soothill J.F. (1978) BMJ 1:
    1443-1445.
10. Goldman A.S. and Smith C.W. (1973) J. Pediat. 82: 1082-1090.
11. Gothefors L. and Marklund S. (1975) Infect. Immun. 11: 1210-1215.
12. Giles C., Sangster G. and Smith J. (1949) Arch. Dis. Child. 24:
    45-53.
13. Svirsky-Gross S. (1958) Ann. Paediatr. 190: 109-115.
14. Tassovatz B. and Kotsitch A. (1961) Ann. Paediatr. 8: 285-288.
15. Smith H.W. (1976) Ciba Symposium 42, "Acute Diarrhoea in
    Childhood", Elsevier Amsterdam, pp 45-64.
16. Jones G.W. and Rutter J.M. (1974) Am. J. Clin. Nutrition 27:
    1441-1449.
17. Rutter J.M., Jones G.W., Brown G.T.H., Burrows M.R. and
    Luther P.D. (1976) Infect. Immun. 13: 667-676.
18. Nagy L.K., MacKenzie T. and Bharucha Z. (1976) Research in
    Veterinary Science 21: 132-140.
19. Nagy L.K., Bhogal B.S. and MacKenzie T. (1976) Res. Vet. Sci.
    21: 303-308.
20. McNeish A.S., Fleming J., Turner P. and Evans N. (1975)
    Lancet 2: 946-948.
21. Stoliar O.A., Pelley R.P., Kaniecki-Green Klaus M.H. and
    Carpenter C.C.J. (1976) Lancet 1: 1258-1261.
22. Smith H.W. (1972) J. Med. Microbiol. 5: 345-353.
23. Kohler E.M. (1974) Am. J. Vet. Res. 35: 331-338.
24. Bullen J.J., Rogers H.J. and Griffiths E. (1978) Current Topics
    in Microbiology and Immunology 80: 1-35.
25. Griffiths E. and Humphreys J. (1978) Eur. J. Biochem. 82:
    503-513.
26. Griffiths E., Humphreys J., Leach A. and Scanlon L. (1978)
    Infect Immun. 22: 312-317.
27. Rogers H.J. and Synge C. (1978) Immunology 34: 19-28.
28. Griffiths E. and Humphreys J. (1977) Infect. Immun. 15: 396-401.
29. Delachaume-Salem E. and Sarles H. (1970) Archives Francaises
    des Maladies de l'Appareil Digestif 59, Suppl 2, pp 135-146.
30. Samson R.R., Mirtle C., McClelland D.B.C. (1979) Immunology
    38: 367-373.

31. Hill I.R. and Porter P. (1974) Immunology 26: 1239-1250.
32. McNeish A.S. (1976) Ciba Symposium 42, "Acute Diarrhoea in Childhood", Elsevier, Amsterdam, pp. 190-192.
33. Steele E.J., Chaicumpa W. and Rowley D. (1974) J. Infect. Dis. 130: 93-103.
34. Heddle R.J. and Rowley D. (1975) Immunology 29: 197-208.
35. Masson P. (1970) "La Lactoferrine", eds Arscia S.A., Brussels.
36. Pitt J., Barlow B. and Heird W.C. (1977) Pedia. Res. 11: 906-909.
37. Fletcher J. (1971) Immunology 20: 493-500.
38. Stephens S., Harkness R.A. and Cockle S.M. (1979) Brit. J. Exp. Path. 60: 252-258.
39. Reiter B., Marshall U.M.E., Bjorck L. and Rosen G. (1976) Infect. Immun. 13: 800-807.
40. Bullen C.L. and Willis A.T. (1971) BMJ 3: 338-343.
41. Dolby J.M., Stephens S. and Honour P. (1977) J. Hyg. Camb. 78: 235-242.

INFANT FEEDING AND THE FAECAL FLORA

C.L. Bullen

The Old Rectory
Fulletby
Nr. Horncastle
Lincolnshire, U.K.

The type of milk fed to newborn infants greatly influences the physio-chemical and microbiological properties of their faeces. Breast-fed babies are relatively resistant to gastroenteritis[1,2,3]; various explanations suggested for this include passive transfer of antibodies to Escherichia coli in colostrum[4,5], contamination of artificial feeds during preparation[6] and the nature of the intestinal environment[2]. The continuing occurrence of enteropathogenic E. coli infections in infants, together with the introduction of "humanised" milks and the popularity of supplementing breast feeding with cows' milk preparations during the first week of life, has led us to re-examine this problem.

From in vitro studies of breast-fed infants, a number of factors seem likely to influence the establishment and maintenance of the bifidobacterial flora and low pH characteristic of the faeces of young infants. There may be specific factors in human milk that either encourage the growth of bifidobacteria or suppress that of E. coli. Breast milk contains a factor that is essential for the growth of one strain of lactobacillus[7]. The addition of lactulose to modified cows' milk preparations induces a predominance of lactobacilli in the faeces of infants[8,9], but this is not accompanied by a consitently low pH. The high content of iron-binding proteins, predominantly lactoferrin, in human milk can inhibit E. coli[10,11]. Lactoferrin in combination with specific antibody to E. coli has a powerful bacteriostatic effect that is abolished when the lactoferrin is saturated with iron.

The results of earlier studies[12] are in general agreement with the observations and conclusions of Ross and Dawes[2]. Breast-fed infants produce an acidic environment in the lumen of the large intestine, and acetic acid is frequently present as an acetate buffer[13]. In vitro experiments suggest that such a buffer exerts a bacteriostatic effect upon Gram-negative and putrefactive organisms[14]. Although we do not exclude the possible role of other specific factors, our findings point to the importance of the ingredients and properties of breast milk, which seems to provide an intestinal content that is favourable both for the growth of bifidobacteria and for the production of an acid environment.

We decided therefore to investigate the microbiological and physiochemical properties of the faeces from infants fed (1) breast milk only, (2) "humanised" milks i.e. cows' milk preparations with the protein and carbohydrate content adjusted to concentrations similar to those of breast milk and with buffering capacities only slightly greater than that of breast milk, and (3) breast milk supplemented with cows' milk preparations during the first week of life and thereafter breast milk only.

MATERIALS AND METHODS

Test and control feeding groups

The study was carried out with 47 infants; 13 were breast-fed and did not receive a supplement, nine were fed Cow and Gate Premium milk, 10 were breast-fed but received cows' milk supplementary feeding once every 24 hours during the first week of life. Faecal samples were examined once a week from birth to the end of the sixth week for viable bacterial counts, pH and the presence and identity of volatile products of bacterial metabolism; the samples were stored at 4°C before delivery to the laboratory. Various factors prevented us from collecting all the specimens from every infant and in some infants the milk preparation was changed before the sixth week. Consequently the number of infants in the four groups varied from week to week.

Buffering capacity

The buffering capacities of breast milk, Premium milk and Gold Cap milk were measured over the pH range 6.8 to 4 with N/10 lactic acid and a Pye Unicam pH meter. The powdered milks were reconstituted according to the manufacturer's instructions.

Chromatographic analysis

25% aqueous suspensions of faecal material were examined by gas chromatography. The procedure for the analysis of acid products was that recommended by Holdeman and Moore[15], the faecal suspensions being examined before and after acidification, and the volatile fatty acids present, recorded.

Microbiological studies

The pH of 10% faecal suspensions in 0.15 m NaCl was measured, using the Pye Unicam pH meter. Total viable counts were made by the method of Miles, Misra and Urwin[16]; counts for E. coli were made on MacConkey agar; those for the anaerobic bifidobacteria were performed on reinforced clostridium medium (R.C.M.) (Oxoid) solidified with 0.75% of New Zealand agar, at pH 5.0, and containing 0.1% cotton blue. The medium is inhibitory to the growth of E. coli due to its low pH value, and its low agar concentration permits the growth of large colonies (2.5 to 3.0 mm diameter) of bifidobacteria. Counts for the clostridia and bacteroides were performed upon Columbia agar (Oxoid) containing 100 µg/ml of neomycin sulphate and 7% horse blood. The anaerobic atmosphere contained 10% CO_2. Viable counts were made on the aerobic plates after 24 hours incubation at 37°C, and on the anaerobic plates after 48 hours. Counts for other aerobes were performed on blood agar.

RESULTS

STUDIES ON MILK PREPARATIONS

Composition of Premium, Gold Cap and breast milks

Table 1 shows the concentrations of fat, protein, carbohydrate and phosphorus in breast milk, and in Premium and Gold Cap milk reconstituted as recommended by the manufacturer.

Table 1

Ingredients	Concentration (g per 100 ml) of the stated ingredient in		
	Cow and Gate Premium milk*	S.M.A. Gold Cap milk*	breast milk[†]
Fat	3.3	3.6	4.6
Total protein	1.8	1.5	1.3
Casein	0.57	0.6	0.4
Soluble Protein	1.23	0.9	0.9
Carbohydrate	6.9	7.2	6.9
Phosphorus	0.04	0.044	0.013

* Figures compiled mainly from manufacturers' current products information.
[†] Figures compiled from Oser (1965)

Buffering capacity

The ratios of the buffering capacities of breast, Premium and
Gold Cap milks were 1.0 : 1.6 : 1.9.

STUDIES ON FAECES

Macroscopic appearance of faeces

Stools from the breast-fed babies were of small bulk, with a
watery curdled consistency, yellow-green colour, and "cheesy" odour.
In the first week, the stools of the bottle-fed infants bore a
resemblance to those of the breast-fed infants; they had a slightly
"cheesy" odour and contained curds, but the number of motions passed
was less and the stools were larger and firmer. After the first
week, the stools of bottle-fed babies became putrid and were of a
firm putty-like consistency. The stools from the infants fed
supplemented breast milk appeared identical to those of the breast-
fed infants but they did not develop a "cheesy" odour for several
weeks.

Acetate buffer in the faeces

The faecal material from breast-fed infants produced a chromatographic pattern that showed a striking increase in the acetic acid
content after acidification with sulphic acid (Fig. 1). Faecal
material from artificially fed infants produced a chromatographic
pattern in which no acetic acid was present before acidification,
but a variety of volatile fatty acids appeared after adidification
(Fig. 2). The acetate buffer was present in the faeces of more than

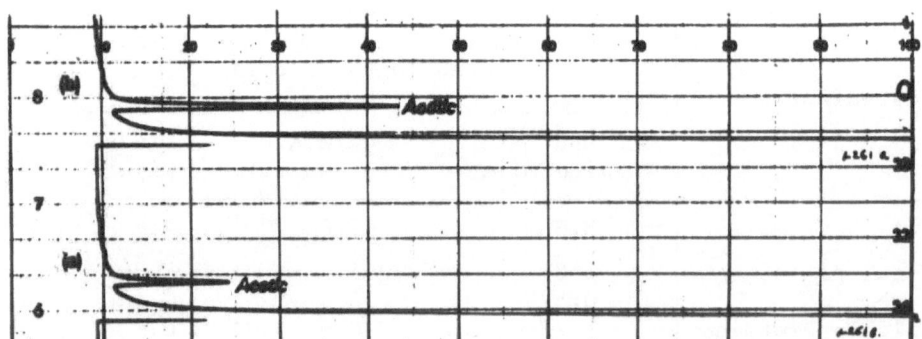

Fig. 1. Chromatograms of the faeces of a breast-fed infant
         (a) acetic acid before acidification of the suspensions,
         and (b) acetic acid after acidification. The difference
         between the two curves represents the presence of acetate
         in the original sample.

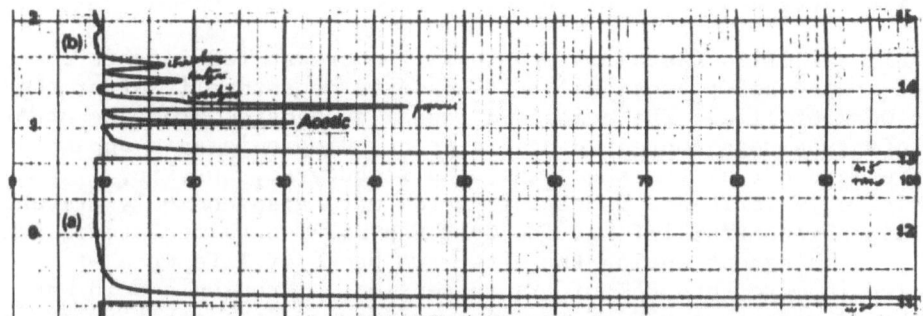

Fig. 2. Chromatograms of the faeces of a bottle-fed infant.
         (a) acetic acid was not present before acidification of
         the suspension, but (b) acetic acid and other volatile
         acids were present after acidification.

60% of the breast-fed infants during the first five weeks of life,
and in 50% in the sixth week. At no time was an acetate buffer
demonstrated in the faeces of the Premium-fed infants. The infants
fed Gold Cap milk did not produce acetate buffer in their faeces
until the fifth and sixth weeks, when a buffer was detected in 16%
and 32% respectively. Of those infants fed breast milk plus
supplement, 20% produced a buffer in the first week, 11.5% in the
second, and 60% in the fourth (Fig. 3).

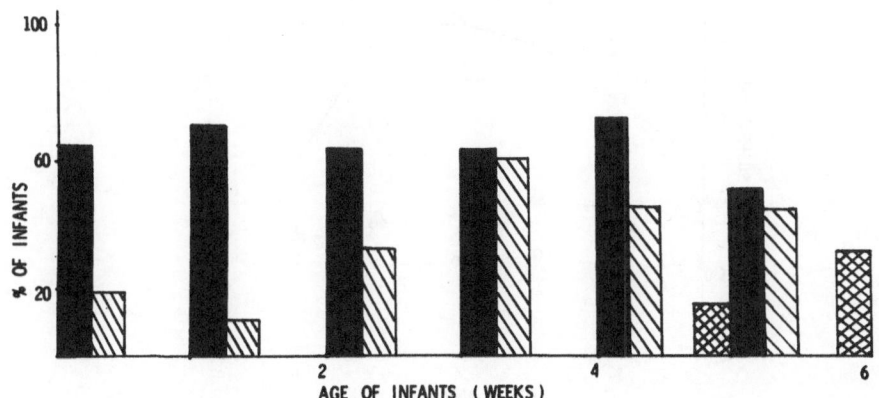

Fig. 3. The presence of an acetate buffer in the faeces of infants
         in the first 6 weeks of life. ■ = breast-fed infants;
         ▨ = infants fed breast milk plus supplement; ▩ = infants
         fed Gold Cap milk.

Volatile fatty acids in the faeces

All acidified faecal suspensions from breast-fed infants contained acetic acid; propionic acid appeared occasionally after the
first week of life. The acidified faecal suspension from the Premium-
fed infants always contained acetic acid. Propionic acid appeared
in more than 83% of the specimens, and isobutyric, butyric,
isovaleric, valeric and isocaproic acids were also commonly present.
The suspensions from infants fed Gold Cap milk contained acetic acid
at all times except during the first two weeks of life when it
appeared in more than 85% of the suspensions. Propionic acid was
present in more than 62% of the suspensions, and the other volatile
fatty acids were also frequently present. In the first week, 71.4%
of the infants fed breast milk plus supplements had propionic and
butyric acids in addition to acetic acid in their faeces. In the
third week, 7.6% of the infants had isobutyric and isovaleric acids
also, but by the sixth week all acids had disappeared except for
acetic and propionic acids. In all infants the occurrence of volatile
fatty acids in the faeces became more frequent during the first three
weeks of life. Table 2 shows the distribution of volatile fatty
acids in the faeces of the four groups of infants during the first
week of life.

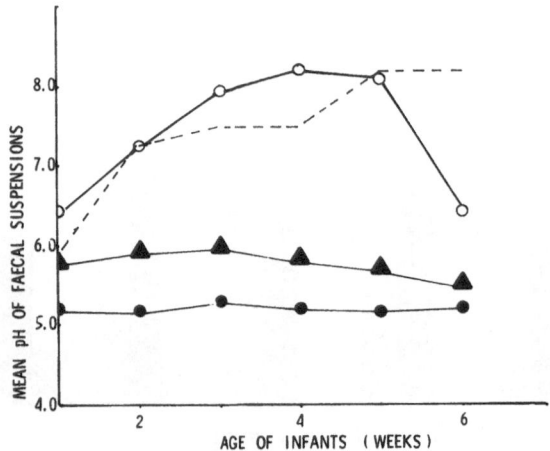

Fig. 4.   Mean pH of faecal suspension from breast-fed infants
          (●————●), infants fed breast milk plus supplement (▲————▲),
          infants fed Cow and Gate Premium milk (–––––), and
          infants fed S.M.A. Gold Cap milk (o————o).

Table 1

Type of food	Number of infants that provided the faecal sample	Percentage of faecal samples in which the stated volatile fatty acids were found							
		Acetic	Propionic	Isobutyric	Butyric	Isovaleric	Valeric	Isocaproic
Cow and Gate Premium milk	8	100	100	25	25	25	0	12.5
S.M.A. Gold Cap milk	8	87.5	62.5	50	62.5	37.5	12.5	12.5
Breast-milk	10	100	0	0	0	0	0	0
Breast-milk plus supplement	7	100	71.4	0	71.4	14.2	0	0

The pH of faeces

Faecal specimens from breast-fed infants were of pH 5.1 to 5.4 throughout the six weeks. In the two groups of bottle-fed infants, the values were in the range pH 5.9 to 7.3 during the first two weeks of life; from the second to the fifth week the pH was in the range 7 to 8.2, but after the fifth week the pH of faecal suspensions from infants fed Gold Cap milk fell to 6.4. In infants fed breast milk plus supplement the neam pH was 5.7 to 6.0 during the first four weeks, falling to 5.45 by the sixth week (Fig. 4).

MEAN VIABLE BACTERIAL COUNTS OF FAECES

Breast-fed infants

From the first week of life there was a marked predominance of bifidobacteria over coliform bacilli and streptococci. Counts of bacteroides were less than 10^8 per g. Counts of clostridia (Clostridium perfringens and Clostridium paraputrificum) rarely exceeded 10^3 per g of faeces, and at times these organisms were not found (Fig. 5a).

Infants fed Premium milk

In the first week of life, bifidobacteria gave a count of more than 10^9 per g of faeces and were predominant over all other bacteria. By the second week, however, the counts of coliform bacilli, strepto- cocci and bacteroides had risen to values of more than 10^9 per g., which were sustained during the six week period; no organism pre- dominated. Viable counts for C. perfringens and C. paraputrificum rose sharply from less than 10^5 per g in the first week of life to more than 10^7 per g in the second and they remained at this level (Fig. 5b).

Infants fed Gold Cap milk

For the first three weeks of life the counts of bifidobacteria, coliform bacilli and streptococci were 10^8 to 10^9 per g of faeces. In the fourth week the coliform bacilli predominated reaching counts slightly above 10^9 per g, whereas the counts of bifidobacteria dropped to 10^7 to 10^8 per g. From the fourth week to the sixth week the coliform counts remained above those of all other bacteria. At no time did the counts of bacteroides fall below 10^6 per g. The counts of C. perfringens and C. paraputrificum rose steadily from 10^5 to 10^6 per g in the first week of life to more than 10^7 per g in the fifth week (Fig. 5c).

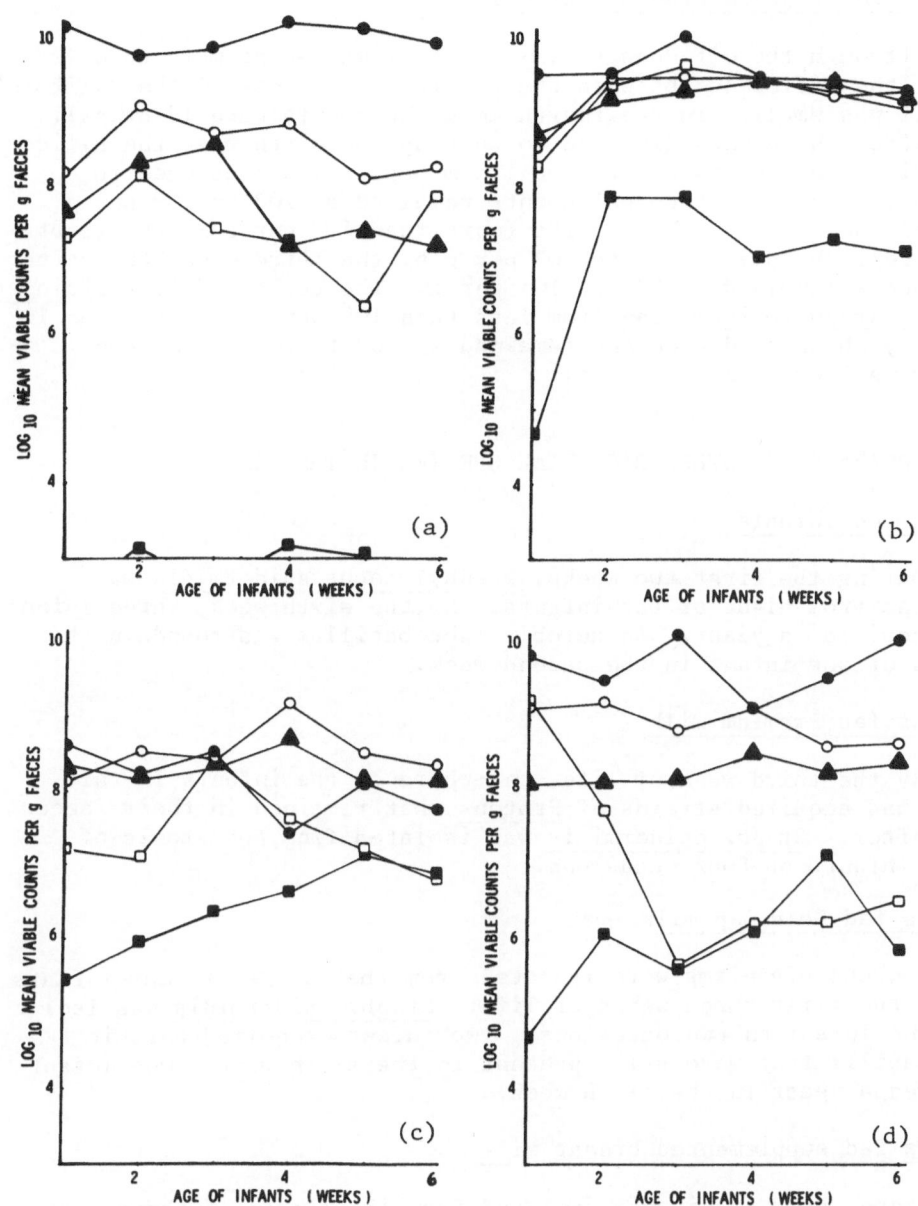

Fig. 5.   Mean viable counts of faecal organisms isolated from
          (a) 13 breast-fed infants, (b) 9 infants fed Cow and Gate
          Premium milk, (c) 10 infants fed S.M.A. Gold Cap milk, and
          (d) 15 infants fed breast milk plus supplement.   ●——● =
          bifidobacteria; o——o = coliform bacilla; ▲——▲ = strepto-
          coccus faecium; □——□ = baceroids; and ■——■ = clostridia.

Infants fed supplemented breast milk

Although the bifidobacterial counts remained at more than 10^9
per g, the difference between their values and those of the coliform
bacilli was small. In the fourth week the counts were identical.
Thereafter the counts diverged so that by the sixth week the bifidobacteria predominated and the coliform population continued to
decrease. The streptococcal counts remained at 10^8 to 10^9 per g
whereas the counts of bacteroids (more than 10^9 per g in the first
week) fell sharply to 10^5 to 10^6 per g by the third week; thereafter
the counts remained at 10^6 to 10^7 per g. The counts of C. perfringens
and C. paraputreficum rose from less than 10^5 per g to more than 10^6
per g by the second week and remained at 10^5 to 10^7 during the
following four weeks (Fig. 5d).

THE APPEARANCE OF OTHER BACTERIAL SPECIES IN THE FAECES

Breast-fed infants

During the first two weeks, staphylococus epidermidis was
cultured from eight of the infants. By the sixth week, three infants
had acquired a yeast. An aerobic lactobacillus was found in the
faeces of one infant in the second week.

Infants fed Premium milk

By the third week of life, one-third of the infants in this
group had acquired strains of Proteus that remained in their faeces
thereafter. Staph. epidermidis was isolated from the stools of
three infants on four occasions.

Infants fed Gold Cap milk

Proteus organisms were isolated from the faeces of four infants
during the first three weeks of life. Staph. epidermidis was isolated
from one infant on two occasions. Two infants acquired aerobic
lactobacilli that were still present in the sixth week. One infant .
acquired a yeast in the sixth week.

Infants fed supplemented breast milk

Staph. epidermidis was isolated from the faeces of three infants
at some time during the six weeks. One infant acquired a yeast in
the third week. Two infants had acquired an aerobic lactobacillus
by the second week. Strains of Proteus were isolated from three
infants by the fourth week, and a strain of Pseudomonas was recovered
from one infant in the third week.

DISCUSSION

The results obtained from this survey support the conclusions reached in earlier feeding trials[17,18] that an important factor that restricts the growth of the Enterobacteriaceae, streptococci, clostridia and bacteroides in the gut of breast-fed infants is the accumulation of acetic acid in the form of an acetate buffer. The primary factor required to ensure acidic faeces is food of poor buffering capacity. The amounts of insoluble protein and phosphorus in the two cows' milk preparations studied in this trial are greater than those present in breast milk; the greater buffering capacities of "humanised" milks reflect their higher content of phosphoro-protein complex. The faeces of infants fed Premium and Gold Cap milks quickly acquire a pH of more than 6.2, and at such a pH an acetate buffer is unlikely to operate. It is interesting that the pH of the faeces continued to rise in these infants, whereas the pH values of faeces from the breast-fed group deviated by no more than 0.2 pH unit throughout the first six weeks of life.

The chromatographic patterns of acidified faecal suspensions from many of the infants fed the two artificial milk preparations showed the presence of a variety of volatile fatty acids. This is in sharp contrast to the patterns produced by the faeces from breast-fed infants in which fatty acids other than acetic acid were rarely present. An acetate buffer was demonstrated in more than 60% of wholly breast-fed infants in the first four weeks of life, whereas infants fed Premium and Gold Cap milks did not produce any buffer and the patterns of volatile fatty acids are reflections of the mean viable counts of the organisms isolated from faeces. Thus breast milk produced a fermentative flora, whereas Premium milk, which has a greater buffering capacity than that of breast milk, produced a putrefactive flora, although the counts of bifidobacteria were high. This suggests that the buffering capacity of the food was sufficiently low to encourage the growth of bifidobacteria, but too high to allow an accumulation of acetic acid in the faeces. Gold Cap milk, however, which has a buffering capacity almost twice that of breast milk, produced a typical putrefactive faecal flora similar to that of a bottle-fed group of infants[13]. A consistent relationship has not been formed between high counts of bifidobacteria and low counts of E. coli in the stools of newborn infants fed breast milk or artificial milk[18]. This was not surprising as none of the infants was wholly breast-fed and only a single observation (at about the seventh day) was made from each individual. Our studies show that breast-fed infants who receive supplements behave as bottle-fed babies. Moreover, the extablishment and subsequent development of the faecal bacterial flora is a dynamic and continuing process that cannot be assessed from a single specimen, especially when such a specimen is taken as early as the seventh day.

The results of the present survey endorse earlier findings[12,13] that the supplementation of breast feeding with artificial feeds of high buffering capacities interferes with the establishment of a fermentative bacterial flora in the gut of the newborn infant, and consequently with the development of acidic faeces. The mean pH of the faeces from the supplement-fed infants was within the acid range, but even after six weeks of life the pH was not as low as that of the faeces of breast-fed infants. This was reflected in the slow appearance of an acetate buffer in the supplement-fed infants; it was not until the fourth week that 60% of these babies had an acetate buffer in their faeces, whereas more than 60% of the breast-fed group produced a buffer within the first week of life.

The chromatographic patterns of volatile fatty acids produced in the faeces of supplement-fed infants indicated an initial putrefactive flora that gradually changed to a fermentative one. When the feeding sequence was changed from a supplemented regimen to breast-feeding alone the subsequent faecal changes took several weeks to develop. The mean viable bacterial counts in the faeces of infants fed supplement reflected the physiochemical changes that occurred. After four weeks of life when, except for acetic acid, the volatile fatty acids were disappearing from the faeces, the bifidobacteria were increasing and gradually came to predominate.

In infants fed only breast milk a strongly acidic environment is produced in the large intestine within the first few days. At the same time, protection is afforded by the bacteriostatic effect of lactoferrin in combination with specific antibody to E. coli[10,12]. As suckling continues, this protection is reinforced and ultimately replaced by that of the acidic environment in the large intestine. It is important to emphasise that when supplements were fed during the first seven days of life the production of a strongly acidic environment was delayed and its full potential was never reached.

ACKNOWLEDGEMENTS

I am indebted to Dr A.T. Willis for his encouragement and advice. I thank Mr P.V. Tearle for the many excellent chromatographic patterns that he provided. I am grateful to Mr J. Harrison for the photographic reproduction of the figures, and to Mrs J. Burton for secretarial assistance.

REFERENCES

1. Alexander M.B. (1948) BMJ 2: 973.
2. Ross C.A.C. and Dawes E.A. (1954) Lancet 1: 994.
3. Hinton N.A. and MacGregor R.R. (1958) Can. Med. Ass. J. 79: 359.
4. Sussman S. (1961) Pediatrics, Springfield 27: 308.
5. Michael J.G., Ringenback R. and Hottenstein S. (1971) J. Infect.
        Dis. 124: 445.

6.   Neter E. (1959) J. Pediat. 55: 223.
7.   Gyorgy P. (1953) Pediatrics, Springfield 11: 98.
8.   Petuely F. and Dristen G. (1949) Ann. Pediat. 172: 183.
9.   MacGillivray P.C., Finaly H.V.L. and Binns T.B. (1959) Scott.
       Med. J. 4: 182.
10. Bullen J.J., Rogers H.J. and Leigh L. (1972) BMJ 1: 69.
11. Bullen J.J., Rogers H.J. and Griffiths E. (1974) in "Microbial
       Iron Metabolism" ed. Neilands J.B., New York, p. 517.
12. Bullen C.L. and Willis A.T. (1971) BMJ 3: 338.
13. Bullen C.L., Tearle P.V. and Willis A.T. (1976) J. Med.
       Microbiol. 9: 325.
14. Bullen C.L. and Tearle P.V. (1976) J. Med. Microbiol. 9: 335.
15. Holdeman L.V. and Moore W.E.C. (1972) Anaerobic laboratory
       manual, Virginia Polytechnic Institute, and State University
       Anaerobe Laboratory, Blacksburg.
16. Miles A.A., Misra S.S. and Irwin J.O. (1938) J. Hyg. Camb. 38:
       732.
17. Willis A.T., Bullen C.L., Williams K., Fagg C.G., Bourne A. and
       Vignon M. (1973) BMJ 2: 973.
18. Hewitt J.H. and Rigby J. (1976) J. Hyg. Camb. 77: 129.

BREAST FEEDING AND VIRUS INFECTIONS

David Tyrrell

Clinical Reserach Centre and
Northwick Park Hospital
Harrow

Every student of medicine and biology is told that the composition of milk is perfectly adapted to the nutritional requirements
of the young mammal and a well fed animal is in many ways no doubt
well able to deal with infections including those due to viruses.
Indeed malnutrition is believed to be an important reason for the
high mortality from measles and herpes simplex virus infections which
occur in certain areas of the world, although this effect is not
independent of immune processes since it is probably due in part to
the lack of immune response in the undernourished infant. Nevertheless good nutrition does not confer immunity against viruses.
In animal husbandry it is well known that animals that are well fed
artificially, especially those deprived of colostrum, are prone to
scours, that is to gastroenteritis, which we now know is often due
to infection with viruses, such as coronaviruses, for example transmissible gastroenteritis (TGE) virus of piglets, and rotaviruses of
piglets, calves and lambs. In such cases it seems that the colostrum
contains antiviral antibodies because the mother has been infected
earlier in life, and these confer resistance to infection with these
viruses[1]. Secretory antibodies are also produced by the respiratory
and gastrointestinal tract and clearly have an important role in
protecting them against infection, but the infant produces these
only later in life and after it has received an antigenic stimulus.

It is unwise however to argue for the value of human milk by
analogy with domestic animals since the anatomy and physiology of
placentation and lactation differ greatly from species to species,
and the pathogenesis of virus infections also varies from virus to
virus. It seems best therefore to review firstly the evidence that
milk, and particularly human milk, has antiviral activity and to
what this may be due. Secondly, we need to review the evidence that

breast feeding actually influences the occurrence of virus infections, for the mere fact that a milk has an antiviral effect against a particular organism in the laboratory does not prove that taking that milk protects the infant to any useful extent against intection with it.

ANTIVIRAL ACTIVITY OF MILK

Antibodies

It is well known that milk contains secretory IgA antibodies, and there is much evidence[2,3] to show that such antibodies directed against the surface antigens of viruses neutralise the infectivity of the virus particle, without the presence of complement or other accessory factors. Although locally administered antigens stimulate particularly high titres of secretory antibodies, human breast milk contains antibody against many viruses to which the mother has been previously exposed, including some which produce localised infections of the respiratory or gastrointestinal tract (Table 1). It is assumed that immunocytes migrate into the mammary gland from other parts of the body where they have encountered antigens[4]. These antibodies are detected most easily in colostrum and decline in concentration as this is succeeded by milk. Thus it seems likely that most children receive maternal antiviral antibody not only via the placenta before birth but also after birth in the milk. Most of these antibodies are believed not to be absorbed but to remain in the intestinal tract after being swallowed, until they are eventually digested. They could therefore be expected to be most effective in preventing infections of the gastrointestinal tract, and it would be unreasonable to expect antibodies against respiratory viruses to be protective even if small amounts of milk were inhaled during suckling.

Table 1. Antiviral antibodies found in human colostrum or milk

Virus	Reference
Polio virus type 1, 2, 3	15
Coxsackie virus types A9, B3, B5	15
Echo virus types 6 and 9	15
Rota virus	7, 16, 17
Respiratory syncytial virus	18
Certain alpha viruses	19

Other antiviral substances

It has been found that milk also has antiviral activity which
is not due to antibodies. For instance, a lipid factor or factors
may have an inhibitory effect on certain arbo viruses[5]. However
we have found that milk can have an antiviral effect on a wide range
of other viruses[6]. The effect is clearly of a different kind from
that produced by antibody and this was recognised as we were
developing a method of assay. To detect antiviral neutralising
antibody it is mixed with a virus and after a delay for reaction the
mixture is added, possibly after dilution, to a system which detects
free virus -- a sensitive tissue culture, for example. If neutralisation has occurred the virus does not infect, and therefore fails to
grow, to damage cells and to cause a cytopathic effect, which is
often detected as a focus or plaque in a cell sheet. This is the
basis of the standard plaque reduction test. Breast milk or fractions
obtained from it can reduce plaque counts of virus even if no specific
antibody is present (Fig. 1), but in this case the virus, the antiviral substance and the cells have all to be present in the same
system and remain together. This suggests that the antiviral substance binds rather weakly to the virus or possibly to the cell.
The antiviral effect is found against a virus such as vesicular
stomatitis virus (VSV) which does not infect man -- nor does any
antigenically related virus -- so an antibody is not likely to be
the explanation (Fig. 1). Furthermore the properties of the activity
do not correspond to those of antibody; for instance it is found
in milk treated with phenol or chloroform-butanol. However it has
not been possible to find a particularly active fraction of human
milk among many provided by Dr G. Spik, and it is difficult to account

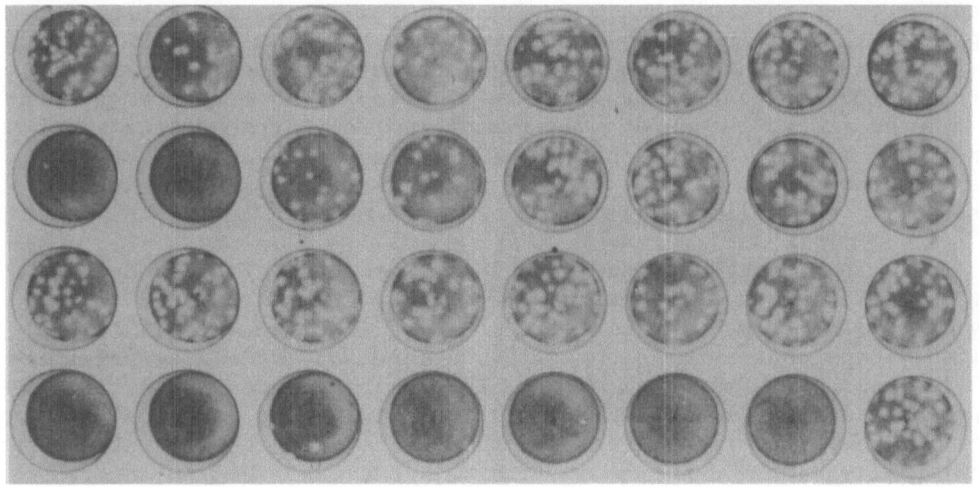

Fig. 1

for all the activity in the original milk from the sum of the
activity of the fractions (K.G. Nicholson, personal communication).
Our present concept is that the effect may be produced by certain
polysaccharides which are found on a number of different molecular
constituents of milk.

Dr Nicholson has also examined samples of breast milk collected
from women in rural Gambia by Dr M. Rowlands and his colleagues.
Some of the results are shown in Table 2 and indicate that although
the activity declines somewhat earlier in lactation it is generally
well maintained thereafter. It may still be present when antiviral
antibody can no longer be detected. Indeed anti rota virus activity
in human milk is probably due to this substrate, particularly later
in lactation[7]. Similar activity is found in cow's milk.

We also studied the effect on breast milk and cow's milk of
various treatments. It was clear that the drying of cow's milk to
produce baby food destroyed much of its antiviral activity, although
pasteurised milk was still antiviral.

Lymphocytes

I include these not because there is much firm knowledge but
because it seems to me to be a subject worthy of exploration.
Lymphocytes sensitised by exposure of the host can be activated and
become transformed by contact with viral antigens. Indeed lymphocyte
transformation is presumably an integral part of the delayed hypersensitivity reaction which seems to make such an important contribution to immunity against viruses such as vaccinia and herpes
viruses[8]. However the question here is whether maternal lymphocytes
contained in colostrum and milk[9] can prevent infection with
respiratory or gastrointestinal viruses. For instance, it has been
suggested that circulating lymphocytes that have not been sensitised
or activated can inactivate viruses if mixed with them. However
further study suggests that the rate of decay of infectivity may not
be reduced in the presence of lymphocytes. Polymorphonuclear cells
can ingest influenza virus particles but are not then infected by
them[9]; they could thus prevent virus particles from attaching to
susceptible epithelial cells.

We also know that lymphocytes in the presence of antibody will
attack cells infected with virus and destroy them (ADCC) and this
may be a means of getting rid of a focus of infected cells. This
antibody dependent cytolysis might take place on the surface of a
baby's mucosa with maternal antibodies and lymphocytes. Most of this
represents nothing more than speculation but it does indicate that
it might be worthwhile trying to develop techniques to separate
functionally active white cells from milk and test them to determine
whether they have antiviral activity. Preliminary evidence shows
that breast milk lymphocytes from 5 of 17 mothers were specifically
transformed by RS virus (Toms G.I., Hey F., Gardner P.S., Pulton C.R.
and Scott R., personal communication).

Table 2. Antiviral activity of Gambian breast milk samples at 20% and 50% concentrations assayed by plaque reduction against vesicular stomatitis virus

Time post-partum	20% milk			5% milk		
	No. of samples	Mean protection	Range	No. of samples	Mean protection	Range
0–2 days	8	85.3	57.1–97.2	8	70.7	48.1–90.5
2–30 days	18	77.7	55.5–97.2	18	47.6	25.3–86.4
1–2 months	14	74.6	55.1–95.1	14	44.6	14.1–80.5
2–4 months	9	71.5	51.8–89.9	9	32.4	19.1–50.4
4–6 months	6	75.1	56.7–83.1	8	36.4	16.6–61.1
6–12 months	4	73.8	52.0–92.9	7	47.8	17.6–68.5
12–18 months	4	63.1	59.5–68.1	7	38.7	9.7–73.3

EVIDENCE THAT BREAST FEEDING PREVENTS VIRUS INFECTIONS

We cannot review here all the evidence that breast feeding reduces the incidence of infections in general in the infant, but apparently the practice reduces the incidence of both gastro-intestinal and respiratory infections[10].

As mentioned earlier it is a most plausible idea that breast feeding may prevent rota virus infections and gastroenteritis. We found in a recent study that rota virus infections were occurring in our area in older children than had been reported by others in previous years in other areas of London[11]. It was known that more mothers in our area were breast feeding their children and for longer than before and it was therefore an attractive hypothesis that this was why the peak age of attack had moved to an older age group. It has been suggested that difficulties in vaccinating successfully with oral polio vaccine are due to prolonged breast feeding as practiced in many tropical countries[12,13]. However the evidence is not con-clusive, and other factors such as infection with other entero-viruses may be more important.

However respiratory disease may also be prevented by breast feeding and recent work in Newcastle has shown that bronchiolitis of infants due to respiratory syncytial virus is less frequent in breast fed than in artificially fed infants[14] (Table 3). The difference remains even when one takes account of the possibility that the effect may be indirect via some secondary association between attitudes to breast feeding and socio-economic status, smoking habits

Table 3. Frequency per cent of breast feeding in patients admitted to hospital in Newcastle with respiratory syncytial virus infections

	R.S. infection		Matched uninfected controls
	all cases	severe cases (tube fed)	
	127	67	497
Not breast fed	30%	28%	49%
Breast fed at time of admission or equivalent age	13%	15%	20%

Adapted from[14].

and so on. The mean relative risk of being in the virus infected
group if the child is not breast fed is 2.2 : 1, although clearly
other factors besides breast feeding probably have some role.

SUMMARY

Breast milk may contain specific neutralising antibodies against
any virus to which the mother has been exposed. It also contains
substances with weak antiviral activity against many viruses. It is
possible that cells present may also have antiviral effects but this
has not been proved. There is some evidence that breast feeding
protects against intestinal infections, for instance with rota
viruses, and also a respiratory virus, namely respiratory syncytial
viruses.

REFERENCES

1. Bachmann P.A. and Hess R.G. in "Virus Infections of the Gastro-
        intestinal Tract", ed. Tyrrell D.A.J. and Kapikian A.Z.,
        Marcel Dekker, New York (in press).
2. Dayton D.H. Jr., Small P.A., Chanock R.M., Kaufman H.E. and
        Tomasi R.B. Jr. (eds.) (1969) "The Secretory Antibody
        System", U.S. Department of Health, Education and Welfare,
        Bethesda, Maryland.
3. Mandel B. (1979) in "Comprehensive Virology 15: Virus-Host
        Interactions; Immunity to Viruses", ed. Fraenkel-Conrat H.
        and Wagner R.R., Plenum, New York and London.
4. Hanson L.Å., Ahlstedt S., Carlsson B., Fällström S.P.,
        Kaijser L.Å., Lindblad B.S., Åkerlund A.S. and Eden C.S.
        (1978) Acta Ped. Scand. 67: 577-582.
5. Falkler W.A. Jr., Diwan A.R. and Halstead S.B. (1975) Arch.
        Virol. 47: 3-10.
6. Matthews T.H.J., Nair C.D.G., Lawrence M.K. and Turrell D.A.J.
        (1976) Lancet 2: 1390.
7. Thouless M.E., Bryden A.S. and Flewett T.H. (1977) BMJ 2: 1390.
8. Goldman A.S. and Smith C.W. (1973) J. Ped. 82: 1082-1090.
9. Hackeman M.M.A., Denman A.M. and Turrell D.A.J. (1974)
        Clinical and Exper. Immunol. 16: 583-591.
10. Robinson M. (1951) Lancet 1: 788-794.
11. Lewis H.M., Parry J.V., Davies H.A., Parry R.P., Mott A.,
        Dourmashkin R.R., Sanderson P.J., Tyrrell D.A.J. and Valman
        Valman H.B. (1979) Arch. Dis. Child. 54: 339-346.
12. Deforest A., Parker P.B., DiLiberti H.H., Taylor Yates H. Jr.,
        Sibinga M.S. and Smith D.S. (1973) J. Ped. 83: 93-95.
13. John T. (1974) J. Ped. 84: 307.
14. Pullan C.R., Toms G.L., Martin A.J., Gardner P.S., Webb J.K.G.
        and Appleton D.R., (1980) BMJ (in press).
15. Michaels R.H. (1965) J. Immunol. 94: 262-271.
16. Simhon A., Yolken R.H. and Mata L. (1979) Acta Ped. Scand. 68:
        161-164.

17. Schoub B.D., Prozesky O.W., Lecatsas G. and Oosthuizen R.
         (1977) J. Med. Microbiol. 11: 25-31.
18. Toms G.L., Pullan C.R., Gardner P.J., Scott M. and Scott R.
         (1980) Arch. Dis. Child. 55: 161-162.
19. Welsh J.K. and May J.T. (1979) J. Ped. 94: 1-9.

FACTORS PREDISPOSING TO FOOD ALLERGY

J.F. Soothill

Institute of Child Health
University of London

Though ill-conceived scepticism is widespread, food allergy is an important cause of disease, and our knowledge of the handling of food antigens results in the perennial doubt -- why do we not all have it? Food antigens are taken up in immunologically considerable quantities (although this is only a very small proportion of what we eat, so digestion and the mucosa are important barriers). Responses occur in all of us to these food antigens -- antibody responses, immune exclusion and partial tolerance -- so the puzzle is not why food allergy occurs, but how do most of us avoid an anaphylactic death after eating food. There are presumable elaborate control systems but since they are poorly understood, their possible defects, which would be expected to contribute to food allergy, are even less clear, but some clinical observations are pointing the way. Allergy, generally, is associated with a range of common minor immunodeficiencies[1], and food allergic subjects take up more food antigen and process it differently (IgG and IgE complexes rather than IgA)[2,3].

SCOPE AND MECHANISMS OF FOOD ALLERGY

Food allergy certainly does occur. Besides clear clinical evidence, the classic passive transfer study of Prausnitz provided clear experimental confirmation years ago. Table 1 lists a number of diseases established to be due to food allergy, by repeated (three times) administration and withdrawal of the food in association with exacerbation and remission of symptoms[4]. Not all food induced symptoms (intolerance) are allergic, however; the non-allergic ones (idiosyncrasy) are largely due to individual enzyme defects (Table 2). It is often difficult to be sure whether a particular sympton is allergic or idiosyncratic, and the two may exist together to the

Table 1. Symptoms securely ascribed to food allergy (especially to cows' milk)

General	Alimentary	Skin	Respiratory	General – secondary to gut allergy
Sudden death	Vomiting	Urticaria	Rhinitis	Failure to thrive
Anaphylactoid collapse	Abdominal pain and distension	Angio-neurotic oedema	Asthma	Anaemia (iron loss)
	Diarrhoea (flat mucosa)	Eczema		Oedema (protein loss)

Table 2

FOOD INTOLERANCE

IDIOSYNCRASY   ALLERGY

Gastrointestinal   Systemic   Gastrointestinal   Systemic
(alactasia)   (phenylketonuria)   (alimentary   (eczema)
                                       cows' milk
                                       allergy)

Table 3. Some foods provoking intolerance

Cow's milk	Meats
Eggs	Cereals
Fish	Yeast
Nuts	Tartrazine, other dyes and preservatives
Pipped fruits	
Shell fish	

same food (e.g. cow's milk protein allergy, and lactose intolerance -- idiosyncrasy). The allergic mechanisms involved in the tissue damage are diverse[5] and are not clearly established. There is evidence for IgE, IgG and complement[6] and T cell mediated ones[7] but their detailed role in different diseases has still to be established and they may well work together. This, and the tendency for atopic subjects to be sensitised to many antigens, only some of which cause symptoms, result in a lack of reliable diagnostic tests, as well as contributing to the doubts about food allergy. Other complicating factors include the fact that, though some symptoms, e.g. local (where it contacts the skin) or systemic or distant (e.g. urticaria or angio-oedema), occur within minutes of contacting the food (presumably at least partly an 'immediate' IgE mediated response), others, such as eczema, may take hours or days to develop so it is difficult for the patient or his parents to note the association between taking the food and getting the symptoms. Also, since many allergic subjects are sensitive to many foods, the avoidance of only some may well not lead to detectable improvement, and the wide use of factory prepared foods, which are usually complex mixtures of antigenic substances (including preservatives and colours, some of which may well provoke idionsyncrasy as well as allergy) often contribute to the diet being unsatisfactory. Because of these difficulties in some patients repeated double blind challenge is needed for diagnostic as well as research purposes[4] and more double blind controlled trials on groups of patients, such as that of Atherton et al[8] which established that eczema is, in fact, food allergy, will be required fully to convince the sceptical. In view of these difficulties, it is important that newer claims for food allergy (behaviour disorders, arthritis) are exposed to similar controlled studies. Scepticism of negative results is also important because it is always possible that the groups are not homogenous and only some of the patients will respond to withdrawal of the foods under consideration, so management of individuals should be guided by repeated double blind studies in them individually. Such studies

will detect intolerance rather than allergy, but it is important
more widely to suspect food allergy, since there is increasing
evidence that we can avoid damaging sensitisation and so prevent
much food allergy, particularly in children in whom it is most
common. It appears that some foods are more allogenic than others;
a list of some common ones is shown in Table 3. But practically all
foods may be allergenic, including such simple substances as the
food dye tartrazine.

FOOD ALLERGY IN ATOPICS

Much food allergy occurs in atopic subjects -- the quarter of
the population which readily develop IgE antibody and so positive
immediate skin responses, to common environmental antigens -- inhalant
and food. This susceptibility is highly familial (more than 50% of
the offspring of atopic subjects are atopic) and antigen-non-specific
-- i.e. an atopic subject will react to many antigens in this way --
but it is unlikely that by no means all the symptoms the atopic
subject suffers from are IgE mediated. Some food allergy occurs in
non-atopics; coeliac disease, a familial vulnerability to a particular
antigen -- gluten -- not associated with atopy, is clearly not IgE
mediated, and is probably T cell mediated[7]. Also, all of us make
IgE, the significance of which is uncertain. The recent report[9]
that non-atopic subjects with migraine have slightly raised levels
of IgE antibodies to the foods which provoke their symptoms (including
such foods as cheese and chocolate, previously thought to work by
idiosyncrasy) indicates the IgE mediated food allergy may be important
in a wider range of disease and subjects that the atopic ones we
recognise at present. This also indicates that drawing the distinc-
tion between food allergy and idiosyncrasy will be difficult.

PREVENTION OF FOOD ALLERGY

Recognition of the immunodeficiency basis of atopy has been
important in leading to an approach to prevention. Though highly
familial, atopy is not entirely genetic, since the concordance of
atopic symptoms is less than 100% in twins[10]. Since the symptoms,
and especially the food allergy, eczema, starts in early infancy,
this relevant environmental factor must operate, in part, in the
neonatal period. This is supported by the effect of time and place
of birth. Asthma is more frequent in those born in the later autumn
in England[11] , and those children of African origin, living in
England, who were born in England, in contrast to those born elsewhere[12]. Though the relevance of these factors has not been
established for food allergy, the strong association of eczema and
asthma suggests that they may be relevant, and the prevalence of
eczema rose greatly with the introduction of artificial feeding of
infants which also suggests that this was leading to sensitisation[13].

There have been several approaches to elucidating the genetic component in atopy. Though tissue type influences the syndrome[14], and there are reports of abnormality of T cell suppression[15] following the demonstration that IgE production is influenced by T cell suppression, it is difficult to be sure whether the latter are causes or effects. The transience of much childhood allergy, and the observation of a range of allergic symptoms in children with immunodeficiencey led to a hypothesis that this might be a general association; the damaging mechanism may be normal but stimulated by excess contact with the antigen at a stage of vulnerability to damaging sensitisation because another mechanism, which would normally have handled the antigen safely, was defective[14].

A persistent pathological hyper-response of one ordinarily protective mechanism may occur as a result of failure of effective antigen handling by another. For example, IgA, the principle secretory immunoglobulin, performs a major protective role at mucosal surfaces. In IgA-deficient subjects there is an increased frequency of precipitins to food antigens[16]. There was a significantly increased proportion of abnormally low serum immunoglobulins in atopic subjects (greater than 2 SD below the normal mean), especially for serum IgA[17]. However, since many subjects in the atopic group had high values, the means of the atopic group did not differ from those of the controls. Transient immunodeficiency, especially in infancy, is recognised as a cause of frequent infection. A prospective study of newborn offspring of atopic parents showed that before symptoms had developed, those who later became atopic (most developed eczema) had lower IgA levels than those who did not develop symptoms, though the difference between the two subgroups had disappeared by one year[18]. It is likely that the IgA deficiency led to the development of atopic disease since it was present prior to manifest disease. It also strengthens the view that neonatal antigen experience in an immunodeficient host is important for allergic sensitisation.

Other immunodeficiencies also may contribute to the development or aggravation of atopic disease, particularly deficiencies in the antibody-complement-phagocyte pathway. Two common defects have been associated with atopy; a defect in yeast opsonisation (a defect of an undefined component of the alternative pathway of complement which is defective in only 5% of the general population but in about 27% of atopic individuals), and a defect in the second component of complement (low levels are found in about 1.5% of the general population but in about 22% of atopic individuals)[19]. Support for the fact that these defects are primary, that is they are not secondary to atopic disease, comes from the finding that they are virtually exclusive; if in an atopic child one is defective, the other is normal. Many children with a rarer deficiency in neutrophil mobility are atopic[20]. Also, there is a high incidence of atopy in subjects homozygotic or hererozygotic for cystic fibrosis[21]. The association of atopy with this range of defects of functions

strongly suggests that defective antigen handling is a general basis
of atopy. Since food allergy may follow infection in relatively
immunodeficient children[22] it is likely that the mechanism involved
in these interelationships is complicated.

PREVENTION OF FOOD ALLERGY

     The concept of the special vulnerability of some children,
specially in the newborn child, led to attempts at prevention by
feeding. In a retrospective study it was shown that witholding
certain sensitising foods from the mother during pregnancy and
excluding wheat, egg, fowl, and dairy products from the child's diet
for the first nine months of life (the diet was soya based) resulted
in a significant lowering of the incidence of atopic dermatitis[23].
Of the infants on the diet who did develop eczema, only 15% developed
subsequent respiratory allergy compared to 60% of their eczematous
siblings who were permitted a nonrestricted diet from birth. A
subsequent prospective study[24] confirmed this. A prospective
controlled study of an antigen avoidance regimen showed that breast
feeding prevented eczema[25]. This has been confirmed[26,27]. It
has also been shown that asthma may be prevented[27] suggesting that
the effects are not antigen specific, and confined to a response to
the foods avoided.

     Since these effects are not 100% and not all mothers can achieve
complete breast feeding, it is important to elucidate the mechanisms
involved. The responses to ingested antigens are complicated and
are inherited independently. Transient defects and imbalances of
such responses could underlie food allergy, so the benefit would
arise from avoideance of early contact with the food. Support for
this comes from the demonstration that milk from sensitised mother
rats suppresses the subsequent IgE antibody response in an antigen-
specific way[28]. This may indeed be part of the story, but does
not explain the apparent antigen-non-specific effects on responses
to non-food allergens. Further rat studies[29] show, however, that
supplementary feeds to young rats increase the subsequent IgE response
of the offspring in an antigen-non-specific way too.

     These antigen-non-specific effects point to more indirect
mechanisms. Artificially fed babies have an intestinal flora somewhat different from that of breast-fed babies, with a predominance
of E. coli[30]; the effect of immunodeficiency on this is not yet
known, but it may exaggerate the burden of E. coli in the intestinal
tract. An effective way of producing IgE antibodies in an experimental animal is to administer very small doses of antigen (it can
be by mouth) at the same time as a strong adjuvant[28]. E. coli
endotoxin is a powerful adjuvant. It is speculated that the
artificially fed, slightly immunodeficient child may fail to control
the E. coli flora sufficiently so that excessive entry of E. coli

endotoxin acts as a potent adjuvant, resulting in IgE antibody
formation to environmental allergens, food, and other normally
swallowed substances. This could enhance sensitisation to ingested
allergens from food or other sources.

TREATMENT OF FOOD ALLERGY

The principal line of treatment of food allergy is avoidance
of the offending foods. Since much food allergy of early childhood
recovers, the case for investigating more heroic approaches is not
clear. Assertions of benefit from drugs (other than symptomatic
measures in eczema etc.) and hyposensitisation have still to be
confirmed by controlled trial.

REFERENCES

1.   Soothill J.F. (1976) Proc. Roy. Soc. Med. 69: 439.
2.   Paganelli R., Levinsky R.J. et al (1979) Lancet i: 1270.
3.   Brostoff J., Carini C. et al (1979) Lancet i: 1268.
4.   Goldman A.S., Anderson D.W. et al (1963) Pediatrics 32: 425.
5.   Coombs R.R.A. and Gell P.G.H. (1975) page 761 in "Clinical
        Aspects of Immunology, 3rd edition" Blackwells, Oxford.
6.   Matthews T.S. and S-othill J.F. (1970) Lancet ii: 893.
7.   Ferguson A. and Parrott D.M.V. (1973) Transplantation 15: 546.
8.   Atherton D.J., Sewell M. et al (1978) Lancet i: 402.
9.   Monro J., Brosthoff J. et al (1980) Lancet ii: 1.
10.   Van Arsdel P.P. and Motulsky A.G. (1959) Acta Genet. 9: 101.
11.   Warner J.O., Price J.F. et al (1978) Lancet ii: 912.
12.   Smith, Morrison J. (1973) Clin. Allergy 3: 269.
13.   Grulee C. and Sanford H. (1936) J. Ped. 9: 223.
14.   Soothill J.F., Stokes C.R. et al (1976) Clin. Allergy 6: 305.
15.   Juto P. and Strannegard M.D. (1979) J. Allergy Clin. Immunol. 64
        64: (1) 38.
16.   Buckley R.H. and Dees S.C. (1969) N. Engl. J. Med. 281: 465.
17.   Kaufman H. and Hobbs J.R. (1970) Lancet ii: 106..
18.   Taylor B., Norman A.P. et al (1973) Lancet ii: 111.
19.   Turner M.W., Mowbray J.F. et al (1978) Clin. Exp. Immunol.
        34: 253.
20.   Hill H.R. and Quie P.G. (1974) Lancet i 183.
21.   Warner J.O., Norman A.P. et al (1976) Lancet i: 990.
22.   Harrison M., Kilby A. et al (1976) BMJ 1: 1501.
23.   Glaser J. and Johnstone D.E. (1953) J.A.M.A. 153: 620.
24.   Johnstone D.E. and Dutton A. (1966) N. Engl. J. Med. 274: 715.
25.   Matthew D.J., Taylor B. et al (1977) Lancet i: 321.
26.   Chandra R.K. (1979) Acta Paediatr. Scand. 68: 1.
27.   Saarinen U., Kajossaari M. et al (1979) Lancet ii: 163.
28.   JarrettE.E. (1977) Lancet ii: 223.
29.   Roberts S.A. and Soothill J.F. (1980) submitted for publication.
30.   Bullen C.L., Tearle P.V. et al (1977) J. Med. Microbiol.
        10: 404.

REGULATION OF IgE ANTIBODY RESPONSIVENESS BY

INGESTION OF ANTIGEN AND BY MATERNAL INFLUENCE

Ellen E.E. Jarrett

Department of Veterinary Parasitology
University of Glasgow

INTRODUCTION

Most of the antigens which enter the body in any large quantity are food antigens. Nature has provided a mechanism whereby the transition from the shelter of intra-uterine life to the antigenic assault of the outside world is taken gradually. The very young mammal is spared the massive onslaught of food antigens by a suckling period, the duration of which varies from species to species according to the maturity of the animal at birth. It is only civilised man who interferes with this arrangement.

The suckling animal has not necessarily been completely shielded from antigenic experience: food and other antigens are capable of being transferred across the placenta[1,2,3] and in the maternal milk[4,5,6,7,8,9,10,11,12] and most young animals will take the exploratory nibble of other foods long before the time when nutritional necessity dictates. Therefore when the time comes to start eating antigens seriously, the young animal may have experienced many of the antigens in question albeit in relatively small amounts. Might this early antigenic exposure have an immunological function? We know that in a small proportion of infants it may lead to sensitisation for IgE production and to food allergy[9,10,11,12]. But what of the remainder? Is the antigen experienced in such small amounts that it is not even recognised, or alternatively could it cause immunological tolerance or active suppression of IgE responsiveness? We do not know.

We are perhaps rather better equipped to understand what happens
to the older animal when it comes to eat antigens in larger amounts.
I shall review experiments in the laboratory which show that both
stimulation and suppression of IgE responses can result.

Young animals differ from older animals not only in that their
immune system may be immature, but also in being compensated for
this deficit with ready-made immunity acquired from the mother.
This takes the form of antibodies which are transferred across the
placenta or in the milk according to species[13], and of sensitised
cells or their products which reach the fetus or neonate by the
same routes[14]. It has recently become evident that this maternal
influence may profoundly affect the IgE responsiveness of young
animals and I shall review our experiments which have demonstrated
this effect. Finally, I shall attempt to draw these points together
in a discussion of the possible interactions of the various factors
which may influence the early development of the IgE producing and
regulating systems.

ORAL STIMULATION AND SUPPRESSION OF IgE RESPONSES

In laboratory animals, when antigen is administered by mouth on
a single occasion, the produciton of a detectable IgE response seems
to depend on the adequacy of the dose of antigen and on the accompani-
ment of some form of adjuvant treatment.

Anaphylactic sensitivity to bovine serum albumin (BSA) occurs
in mice which have been given 4 mg of this antigen together with
Bordetella pertussis (Bp) adjuvant by stomach tube[15]. Detectable
IgE antibody responses can be evoked by orally administered egg-
albumin (EA) with Bp given by the oral or intraperitoneal
routes[16,17].

The amount of antigen necessary to elicit a response depends
on the inate IgE responsiveness of the strain of animals used.
Thus 10 mg EA was the lowest effective dose in LouM/WSL rats[17]
while in Hooded Lister rats which are sensitive to IgE stimulation
with very small amounts of antigen[18] oral immunisation could be
achieved with as little as 10 μg of this antigen[16].

Adjuvant facilitates the induction of IgE antibodies whether
it is presented to the mucosa or by injection. It seems that adjuvant
is a particularly important component of the stimulus for IgE
induction, more so than for other immunoglobulins, and reports of
IgE synthesis without adjuvant are rare, but a reaginic antibody
response to Penicillin G has been shown in mice which were fed this
drug over a prolonged period[19]. Perhaps the action of an
environmental adjuvant such as a bacterial infection during the
period of antigen feeding initiated the IgE response.

Regardless of whether or not an IgE response occurs as the result of feeding antigen a mechanism for the suppression of IgE responsiveness may be activated and detected by a diminished or absent response to a subsequent immunising stimulus. In rats the IgE response to giant ragweed extract and horse serum can be suppressed by oral treatment with these antigens and the suppression is accompanied by protection from anaphylactic shock[20]. Suppression of an IgE response is more effective when oral treatment is started at one month of age than at two or five months, and small frequent doses of antigen are more effective than larger doses at longer intervals. Both IgE and IgG_1 responses to a parenteral challenge of EA and adjuvant were suppressed in mice which had previously received the antigen without adjuvant by stomach tube. Suppression lasted up to eight weeks after oral sensitisation but waning suppression could be reinforced by further oral exposure to EA[21]. A similar phenomenon has been observed in rats which had received EA in their drinking water prior to challenge[22]. When IgE suppression was induced by the oral consumption of Peyer's patch and spleen lymphocytes the frequency of antigen exposure was found to be more important than the dose for the generation of effective suppressor cells[23]. In mice IgE response to subsequent challenge is suppressed in those which have received oral antigen[24].

In the above experiments the antigen was administered orally in soluble form without adjuvant. An IgE response did not occur. The subsequent challenge which tested for responsiveness therefore had to consist of a known immunogenic stimulus (usually antigen + adjuvant intraperitoneally) in order to demonstrate a suppression of response in the treated animals in comparison with previously untreated control animals.

The IgE response may also be suppressed in an animal which is already producing IgE antibody. Thus we found that in rats which had been immunised by the administration of oral antigen and adjuvant subsequent oral challenge without adjuvant resulted in a secondary IgE response, the magnitude of which was inversely proportional to the priming dose of antigen. The booster response was better with a small than with a large dose of antigen (fig. 1). As little as 10 µg EA was sufficient to stimulate an IgE response in a proportion of rats and most of the remainder had evidently been primed as they produced a marked secondary response on challenge one month later. However, as the primary dose of antigen was increased the secondary response to the subsequent challenge became progressively poorer until, in most of the rats which had received 100 mg EA on the first occasion there was no response at all. Fig. 2 shows the results of another experiment which verified this phenomenon and which also included a second challenge.

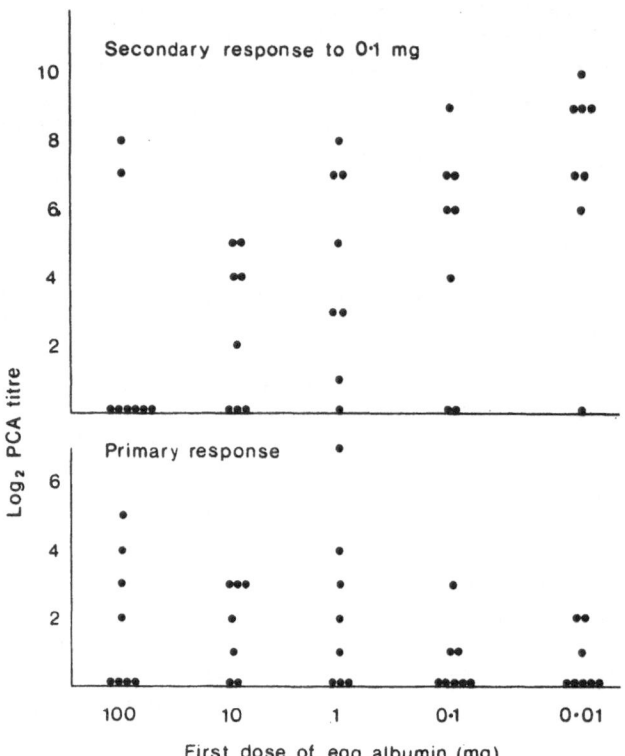

Fig. 1.   IgE response to intragastric egg-albumin. The animals were
immunised with the indicated amounts of antigen administered
by stomach tube. Bordetella pertussis was given by intraperitoneal injection. One month later the rats were
challenged with intragastric antigen, but adjuvant was not
given. The values shown are for the primary IgE responses
on day 12 after immunisation and the booster resonse on
day 4 after challenge. The values for the booster response
are significantly different (p < 0.05) (Kruskal-Wallis
non-parametric analysis of variance (Siegal 1956)). The
figure depicts the results shown in Table 3 of Jarret
et al[16].

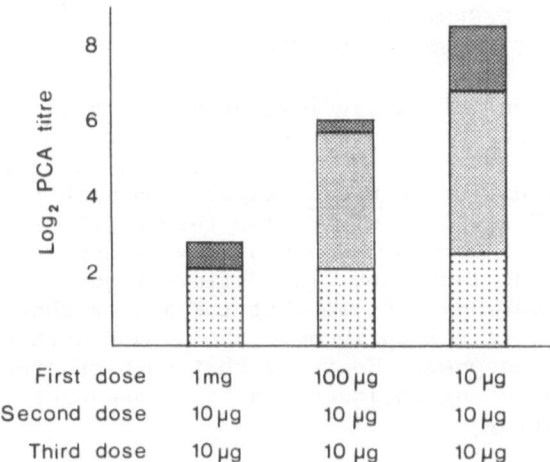

Fig. 2.   IgE response to intragastric egg-albumin. The animals
(6 per group) were immunised with the indicated amounts of
antigen as in the experiment described in Fig. 1, and
challenged one and two months later with 10 µg EA
administered by stomach tube. Shown are the mean EA-PCA
titres 12 days after initial immunisation and the increments
resulting 4 days after antigen challenge. The levels of
both the first and second booster responses are significantly
different (p < 0.02). The figure depicts the results shown
in Table 4 of Jarrett et al (1976)[16].

The immunising stimulus which induces an IgE response can also
activate a counteracting antigen-specific suppressive mechanism.
It is evident that this regulatory mechanism has no effect on the
fully mature antibody-producing cell as the primary response
initiated by the first stimulus is allowed to proceed unhindered
until it eventually fades away. Suppression inhibits the differentiation of the memory B cells which would otherwise be responsible for
the production of a secondary response.

Unfortunately for our present topic the experiments described
above utilised young adult animals. Their relevance to the very
young animal therefore remains to be determined. The young animal
may react quite differently to a similar antigenic stimulus, not only
because of immunological immaturity but also because of the immune
influence of the mother. This latter factor may influence the form
of the response to antigenic stimulation for some time after birth
as is shown below.

SUPPRESSION OF IgE RESPONSIVENESS
IN THE OFFSPRING OF IMMUNISED MOTHERS

Occasionally animals including man may be born hypersensitive
or with specific IgE antibody in the cord blood. As IgE does not
cross the placenta its presence in the neonate indicates fetal
synthesis as a result of in utero stimulation with antigen.
Suppression of IgE response might also result from such an antigenic
stimulus and be more common. Consequently we fed or injected rats
during pregnancy and lactation with different quantities of egg-
albumin (EA) without adjuvant so that the mother should act merely
as a means to passage the antigen to the fetus without herself
producing an IgE response. We found that such treatment of the
mothers did not have any influence on the subsequent IgE responsiveness of the offspring.

These experiments led to others on the effect of immunising
rats with antigen and adjuvant long enough before a pregnancy to
allow the development of an immune response. The prospective mother
rats were immunised with EA and Bp one month before mating. When
the young rats were around six weeks old they were immunised with
EA and Bp and were found to have a greatly depressed IgE response
to EA[25]. This suppression of response is still evident if
immunisation of the offspring is delayed up to fifteen weeks after
birth (unpublished results).

The suppression of IgE responsiveness is antigen specific.
When the offspring of EA immunised or of normal mothers were inocu-
lated with both EA and keyhole limpet haemocyanin (KLH), the IgE
response to EA but not to KLH was depressed in the offspring of the
EA immunised mothers. In order to determine whether the suppressive
effect was transferred transplacentally or by way of the milk, the
offspring of EA immunised and of untreated mothers were exchanged
on the day of birth. The IgE response of these rats following
immunisation at five to six weeks of age was compared with that of
rats reared by their natural mothers. The offspring of normal rats
were suppressed for the IgE response to EA if suckled by previously
immunised mothers while the offspring of immunised mothers fostered
to non-immunised mothers subsequently had a normal IgE response
(fig. 3). This indicated that the factors responsible for
suppression were transferred in the milk. The suppression of
responsiveness is not only antigen specific but also class-selective
(table 1).

It follows that the development of the IgE regulatory mechanism
in the young animal may be influenced by information passed from the
mother. The implication of this finding -- that in nature animals
might be suppressed from birth to the common allergens in the maternal
environment -- remains to be explored, as does the mechanism.

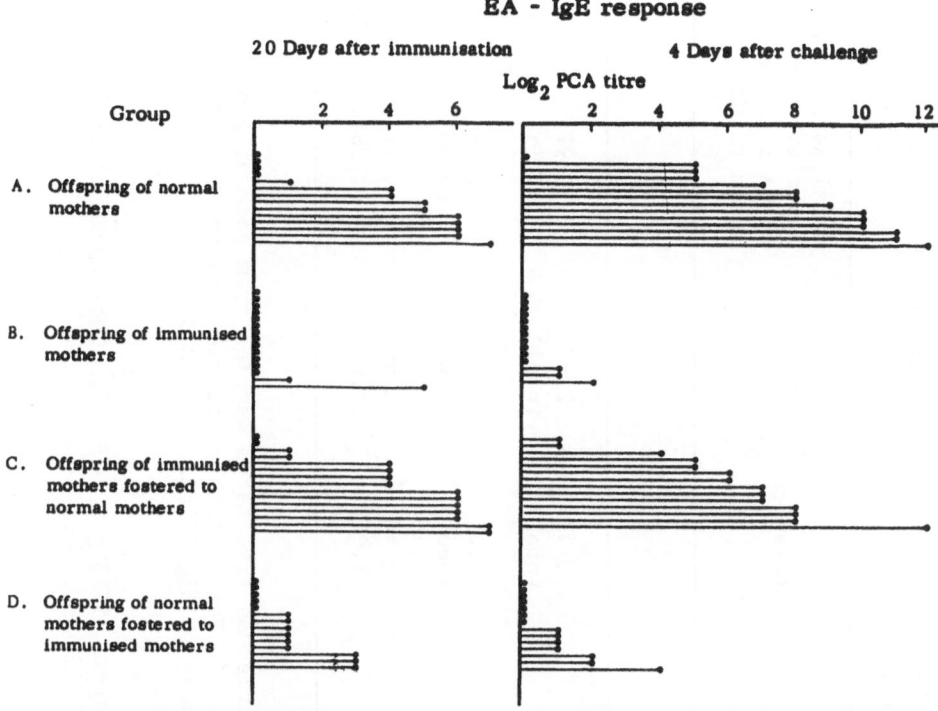

Fig. 3. Selective suppression of IgE antibody responsiveness by
maternal influence: effect of cross-fostering on the
transfer of the IgE suppressive effect. The immunised
mothers were injected with 1 mg EA and 10^{10} Bp one month
before mating; control mothers were untreated. At birth
the offspring were either left with their own mothers, or
were exchanged so that those born of immunised mothers were
suckled by non-immunised mothers and vice-versa. These
exchanges were performed as soon as possible and not more
than one to two hours after birth. Each of the groups A to
D consisted of the female rats of four litters. These rats
were immunised at 5 to 6 weeks with 10 µg EA and Bp and
were challenged one month later with 1 µg EA alone. The
results shown are the primary and booster EA-IgE antibody
responses of individual rats.

ELLEN E. E. JARRETT

Table 1. Comparison of EA-IgG and total antibody response with EA-IgE levels in the offspring of normal (A) and immunised (B) mothers.

	EA-IgE (geometric mean PCA titre)		EA-IgG (mean cmp x 10^{-3}) (± SD)		Total antigen binding capacity (mean $\log_{10}$ µg EA bound/ml serum (± SD)	
	A	B	A	B	A	B
D20 after immunisation	9.18	all negative	1.92 (pool)	2.93 (pool)	0.97 (0.15)	1.35 (0.19)
D4 after challenge	1175	all negative	4.45 (pool)	4.71 (1.43)	1.39 (0.20)	1.47 (0.18)
D21 after challenge	278	all negative	3.39 (1.05)	3.72 (2.62)	1.71 (0.36)	1.49 (0.20)

The measurements shown above were performed on five serum samples from each of groups A and B rats in the experiment illustrated in Fig. 3. The difference between groups A and B on day 20 after immunisation in the antigen binding assay is significant ($p < 0.01$).

DISCUSSION

In adult laboratory animals, the balance of response to administration of antigen, whether by oral or intraperitoneal routes, tends
towards suppression rather than stimulation of IgE production. In
other words the experience of antigen leads more often to a diminished
rather than to a heightened IgE repsonse to another exposure, because
antigen activates not only the precursor cells which will be responsible for antibody production, i.e. IgE B cells and their helper T
cells, but also related supressor T cells which have the function to
regulate that production[26]. A large dose of antigen in the priming
stimulus results in a higher proportion of suppressor T cells in the
primed cell population. Furthermore, a large dose of antigen
especially in the presence of adjuvant stimulates the production of
IgG antibodies which also have a suppressive regulatory effect on
the IgE response[26]. The IgE system appears to be far more
susceptible to suppression than the other immunoglobulin classes.
This makes good biological sense, because whatever the normal function
of IgE, perhaps in the defence against helminth parasites, it is
clearly performed by extremely small amounts, with over-production,
or a response against the 'wrong' antigens leading only to a dele-
terious hypersensitivity. In these terms the absorption of antigen
across mucous membranes in the adult animal is normal and necessary
to maintain the IgE regulatory system in a state of activity.

What may be normal and necessary in the young animal is still
uncertain. Many experiments critical to an understanding of the
situation remain to be done. Meanwhile we can at least consider the
various influences which may contribute to the developing immune
responsiveness of the young animal (fig. 4). First is the variability
inherent in the constitution of the young animal itself; the degree
of immaturity of the immune system at any particular time and the
genetic immune factors which will determine the eventual capacity
of the animal to regulate IgE and other antibody responses. Secondly
there are variables relating to antigen exposure; the molecular con-
figuration, dose, frequency and time of stimulation relative to the
stage of maturity of the animal. Superimposed on these variables
is the influence of the immune response of the mother. The nature
of the messages which the mother will transfer are again determined
by factors under genetic control and by the mother's previous
exposure to antigen. It is unlikely that these various factors will
be found to operate in isolation because each has the potential for
displacing or deforming the effects of the other. It is conceivable
that quite precise interactions, of particular circumstances -- say
the experience of antigen within a certain dose range in the presence
of maternal antibody at a particular stage of immaturity -- may set
the pattern of immune response for life.

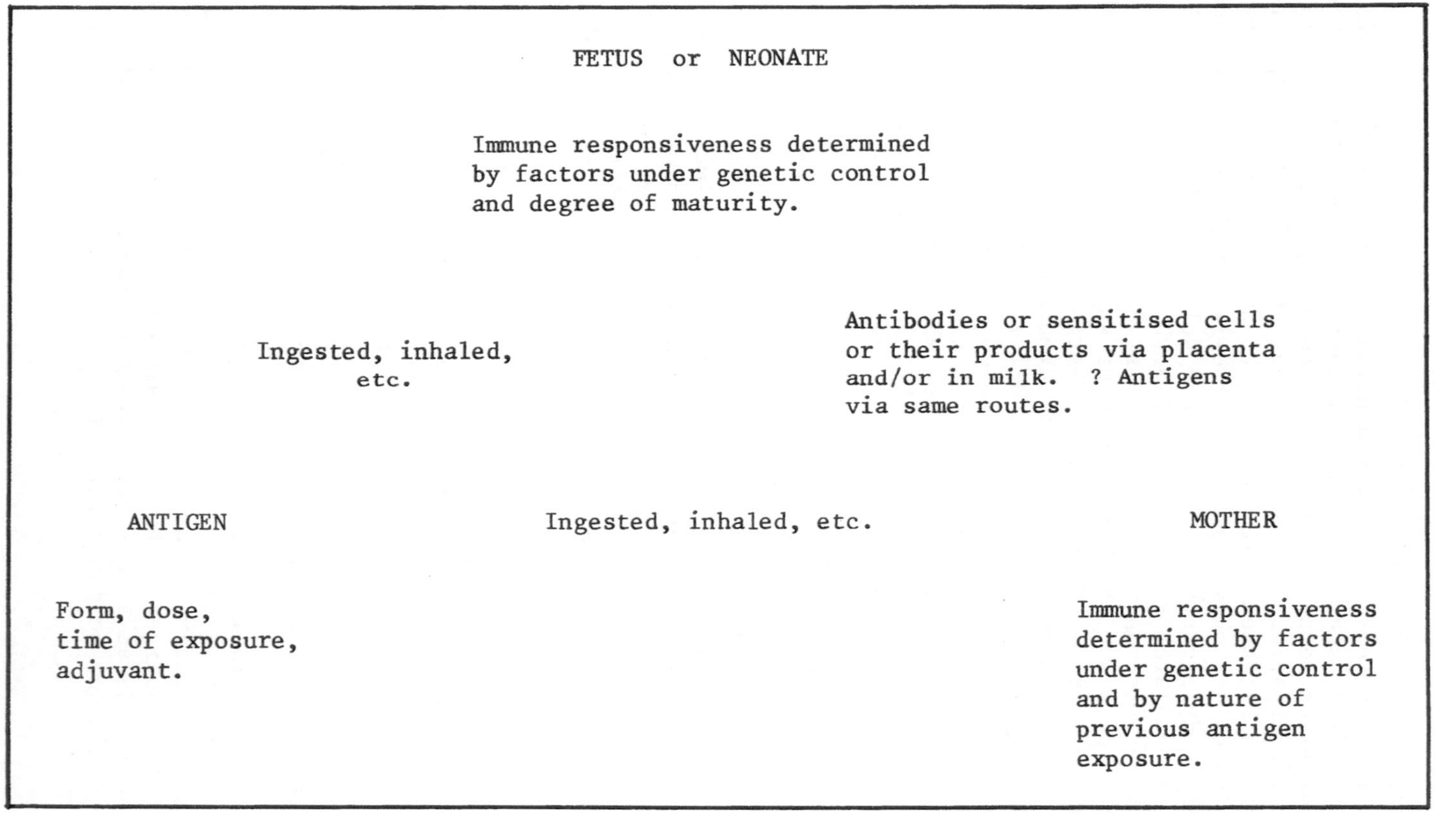

FETUS or NEONATE

Immune responsiveness determined by factors under genetic control and degree of maturity.

Antibodies or sensitised cells or their products via placenta and/or in milk. ? Antigens via same routes.

MOTHER

Immune responsiveness determined by factors under genetic control and by nature of previous antigen exposure.

Ingested, inhaled, etc.

Ingested, inhaled, etc.

ANTIGEN

Form, dose, time of exposure, adjuvant.

Fig. 4. Superimposed variables which may influence the developing immune system of the young animal.

ACKNOWLEDGEMENTS

The work described here was supported by grants from the Medical Research Council, the Wellcome Trust and INSERM (France). The author is a Locke Research Fellow of the Royal Society.

REFERENCES

1. Ratner B., Jackson H.C. and Gruehl H.L. (1927) J. Immunol. 14: 303-319.
2. Kaufman H.S. (1971) Climical Allergy 1: 363-367.
3. Matsumara T., Kuruome T., Oguri M., Iwasaki I., Kanbe Y., Yamada T., Kawabe S. and Negishi K. (1975) Annals of Allergy 35: 221-229.
4. Shannon W.R. (1921) Am. J. Dis. Child. 22: 223-231.
5. Halsey J.F. and Benjamin D.C. (1976) J. Immunol. 116: 1204-1207.
6. Tyrala E.E. and Dodson W.E. (1979) Arch. Dis. Clin. 54: 787-800.
7. Corwell M., Meyer R.R., Pazdermik T.L. and Halsey J.F. (1980) Cellular Immunology 52: 229-283.
8. Kulangara A.C. (1980) I.R.C.S. Med. Sci. 8: 19.
9. Kaplan M.S. and Solhi (1979) J. Allerg. Clin. Immunol. 64: 122-126.
10. Gerrard J.W. (1979) Annals of Allergy 42: 69-72.
11. Jakobsson I. and Lindberg T. (1978) Lancet ii:438-439.
12. Warner J.O. (1980) Clinical Allergy 10: 133-136.
13. Brambel, F.W.R. (1970), "The Transmission of Passive Immunity from Mother to Young", North Holland, Amsterdam (pp. 1-365).
14. Beer A.E., Billingham R.E., Head J.R. and Parmley M.J. (1977) in "Development of Host Defences", eds Cooper M.D. and Dayton D.H., Raven Press, New York.
15. Hof H., Finger H., Kornes C. and Milke C. (1975) Zbl. Bact. Hyg. I Abt. Orig. A. 230: 210-222.
16. Jarrett E.E.E., Haig D., McDougal W. and McNulty E. (1976) Immunology 30: 671.
17. Bazin H. and Platteau B. (1976) Immunology 30: 679.
18. Jarrett E.E.E. and Stewart D.C. (1974) Immunology 27: 365.
19. Perelmutter L. and Liakopoulou A. (1975) Acta Allergol. 30: 250.
20. David M.F. (1977) J. Allerg. Clin. Immunol. 60: 180-187.
21. Vaz N.M., Maia L.C.S., Hanson D.G. and Lynch J.M. (1977) J. Allerg. Clin. Immunol. 60: 180-187.
22. Bazin H. and Platteau B. (1977) Biochem. Soc. Trans. 5: 1571.
23. Ngan J. and Kind L.S. (1978) J. Immunol. 120: 861-865.
24. Hanson D.G., Vaz N.M., Maia L.C.S. and Lynch J.M. (1979) J. Immunol. 123: 2337-2343.
25. Jarrett E.E.E. and Hall E. (1979) Nature 280: 145-147.
26. Tada T. (1975) Prog. Allergy 19: 122-194.

EFFECTS OF MALNUTRITION ON SPECIFIC CELL-MEDIATED

IMMUNE RESPONSES

R.K. Chandra

Memorial Univeristy of Newfoundland
St. John's, Newfoundland
Canada

Nutritional deficiency influences every organ in the body and adverse effects of protein-energy malnutrition on the liver, gastro-intestinal tract, pancreas, brain, skin and mucous membranes have been well described. The association of malnutrition and infection has received increasing attention in the last few years and there have been many comprehensive systematic studies of the influence of nutritional deficiency on both antigen-specific and non-specific immune responses in man and laboratory animals. Moderate to severe protein-energy undernutrition impairs several facets of host resistance. In this selective review the effects of malnutrition on specific cell-mediated immune responses are summarised; other aspects of the nutrition-immunity-infection interactions have been discussed elsewhere and reference should be made to exhaustive reviews[1,2,3,4,5,6,7,8,9].

INFECTIONS IN THE MALNOURISHED

The experience of clinicians and public health professionals working in developing countries has indicated that infections occur more frequently and are more fulminant and lethal in malnourished subjects. Epidemiological data from field surveys in Asia and the Americas have confirmed the intimate association of nutritional deficiencies with the failure of growth and with infections illness, particularly diarrhoeal disease. A Pan American Health Organisation survey of childhood mortality patterns in the Americas showed that 57% of children under five years of age who died showed sign of intrauterine or postnatal nutritional growth retardation as either the primary or an associated cause of death. In a prospective study in Mexican children, followed weekly from birth to five years of age, moderate malnutrition correlated significantly with the duration and

severity of episodes of infectious disease and to a lesser extent
with the incidence of diarrhoeal disease in the age period eight to
eighteen months. The majority of hospitalised children with severe
forms of malnutrition have an associated infection at the time of
admission; this is more often observed in kwashiorkor than in
marasmus.

Measles and other infectious diseases run a more severe course
in nutritionally deprived children. Measles is known to produce
fatal giant-cell pneumonia in children with kwashiorkor. It is
interesting that there is an unexplained geographical difference in
measles-associated morbidity and mortality: the frightening severity
of measles in African infants with kwashiorkor has not been observed
in marasmic Asian children. In kwashiorkor herpes virus infection
is often generalised and fatal adrenal, hepatic, and cerebral
haemorrhages are seen at autopsy and there is a conspicuous lack of
inflammatory response. Septicaemia due to gram-negative microorganisms and respiratory infections caused by pneumonocystis carinii
frequently complicate both primary and secondary moderate-to-severe
protein-energy malnutrition.

Heavier loads of parasites, particularly ascaris lumbricoides,
necator americanus, strongyloides stercoralis, giardia lamblia, and
entamoeba histolytica, are encountered in malnourished groups. This
is not to say that nutritional deficiency necessarily leads to heavy
parasite infestation -- the reverse is probably often true. However
in laboratory animals experimental protein deficiency generally
 acilitates protozoal and helminthic infection. Also, undernourished
persons and small-for-gestation, low-birth-weight infants often show
greater rates of infection with enteropathogens, for instance shigella
spp. The incidence and severity of pneumonia and diarrhoeal disease
is greatly increased, with a consequently higher death rate, and the
detection rate of hepatitis B surface antigen in the serum is several
times higher. Osler's description of the intimate association between
inanition and tuberculosis has been supported by recent data.

The concept of antagonism should be mentioned. There are a few
isolated clinical and experimental observations that point to enhanced
host resistance to some viral infections in moderate undernutrition.
However most data suggest an increased susceptibility of individuals
with protein-energy malnutrition to infectious diseases. This has
been supported by extensive experiments in laboratory animals in
whom nutritional deprivation is almost invariably associated with
increased morbidity and mortality following challenge with a variety
of microorganisms.

Malnutrition is not confined to the Third World. In recent
years there has been increasing recognition of the frequent presence
of protein-energy malnutrition in hospital patients. In such subjects
there is a good correlation between the presence of nutritional

deficiencies on the one hand and sepsis and mortality on the other. In many studies of patients with lymphoreticular malignancies, the occurrence of complicating pneumocystis carinii and other life-threatening infections was related to lower concentrations of serum proteins, especially albumin. This confirmed controlled observations in rats whose susceptibility to pneumocystis carinii infection was enhanced by protein deficiency. The frequency of malnutrition as judged by body weight, skin fold thickness, and the serum albumin concentration in hospital patients in many affluent countries is high, and this is related to their decreased ability to mount a delayed hypersensitivity reaction ot common recall antigens. Post-operative sepsis and mortality can be related to preoperative albumin and transferrin levels and with anergy. Nutritional support may reverse these changes and reduce the incidence of fatal pyogenic infections. These observations suggest that nutritional assessment is useful for selecting those individuals that may be at high risk of developing infection and who would benefit from short-term nutritional supplementation before surgical operation. This is also true of growing infants in the community.

The interaction of specific nutrients and susceptibility to infection should be considered. Whereas there are considerable data on the mutually augmenting effects of PEM and infection, similar information for deficiencies of individual nutrients is not available. This is understandable, since nutritional deficiencies in man are often multiple and each nutrient may exert a variable, possibly even opposing, influence on the occurrence of infection. Some surveys have reported a decrease in the frequency of infection among infants fed iron-fortified milk, whereas others have failed to detect such an association. Iron deficiency has been noted to be a common denominator of chronic mucocutaneous candidiasis and therapy with iron preparations rapidly improved the dermatological lesions and associated immunological changes. An association between a higher frequency of infection and iron-deficiency anaemia has been seen in Indonesian plantation workers; iron supplements decreased the incidence of common gastrointestinal and respiratory infections: unfortunately, concurrent observations were not made in any control groups. A Tanzanian report suggesting a lower frequency of infection in iron-deficient subjects than in those with other types of anaemia has been difficult to interpret because of lack of data on any healthy controls in the same community. In laboratory animals, controlled deprivation of specific nutrients generally increases host susceptibility to pathogens and infection-related mortality[6].

HISTOMORPHOLOGY OF LYMPHOID ORGANS

One of the earliest indications of nutritional effects on immunity was the observation of thymic atrophy in children and adults dying of severe malnutrition, both kwashiordor and marasmus, often complicated by infection. Changes in thymic size may also be seen

on X-ray of the chest in life. Histological examination of the thymus
reveals loss of corticomedullary differentiation, reduction in the
number of lymphocytes and degeneration of Hassal bodies (Fig. 1).
Tonsillar size is often small. Atrophy is also seen in the para-
cortical regions of lymph nodes and periarteriolar cuffs of splenic
vasculature. There is paucity of lymphocytes in these thymus-
dependent areas. Similar changes have been seen in laboratory animals
deprived of protein, energy and various specific nutrients. In these
deficiencies of single nutrients, a reduction in the number of mononuclear cells in the lymphoid organs has been recorded.

DELAYED CUTANEOUS HYPERSENSITIVITY

    Observations in the early 1960s showed that the tuberculin
reaction was often negative in malnourished children with active
tuberculosis. Similarly Mantoux conversion after B.C.G. vaccination
is less often seen in malnourished populations than in healthy, well
nourished controls[11,12]. The delayed cutaneous hypersensitivity

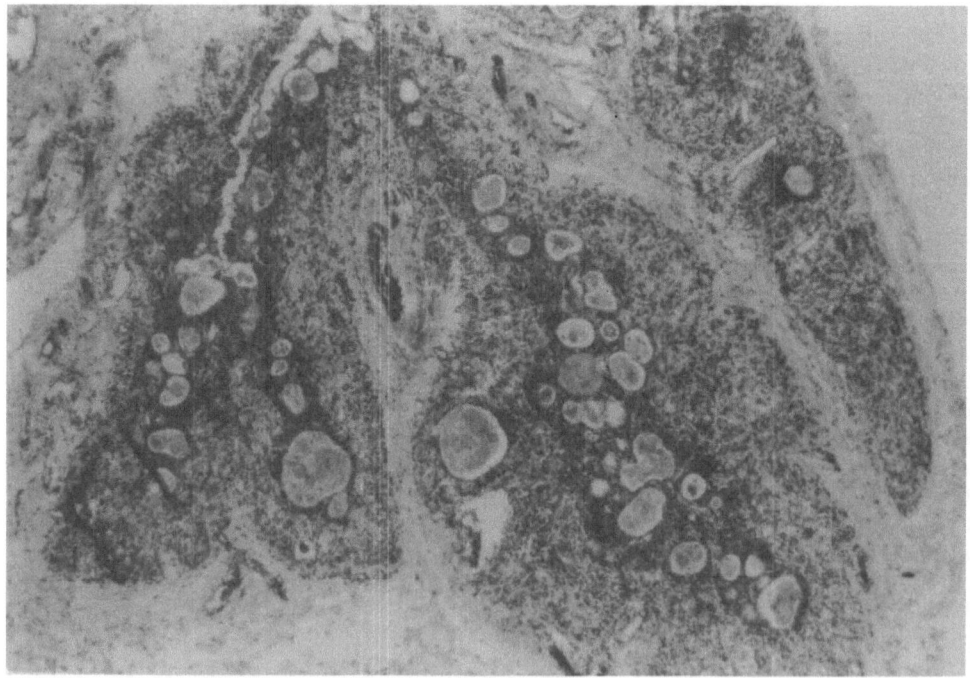

Fig. 1.   Thymus in protein-energy malnutrition. Note paucity of
          lymphocytes and degeneration of Hassal corpuscles.

responses to a battery of ubiquitous recall antigens, candida, streptokinase-streptodornase, mumps and trichophyton have been studied. When a standard dose of the antigen is injected intradermally on the volar surface of the forearm and the diameter of induration read after 48 to 72 hours, both the frequency and the size of the induration are reduced in protein-energy malnutrition (Table 1)[11, 13,14,15]. There could, of course, be a number of underlying mechanisms for such anergy and faults in the afferent and efferent limbs of the immune arc as well as in the central component of antigen recognition and proliferation may be important. Using 2, 4 dinitro-chlorobenzene, it has been observed that both sensitisation and expression may be impaired, the latter partly the result of reduced inflammatory response.

LYMPHOCYTE SUBPOPULATIONS

Thymus-dependent T lymphocytes are recognised by their ability to form rosettes with sheep red blood cells. The number of rosette-forming T lymphocytes is reduced in children with protein-energy malnutrition (Fig. 2)[16,17]. This is true of even those with marginal and moderate deficits of nutrient intake. On the other hand, the proportion of surface Ig-bearing B lymphocytes involved in immunoglobulin synthesis is unchanged. Thus we are left with a large number of circulating lymphocytes that do not bear the conventional surface markers of either T or B cells; these cells have been called the "third population" or "null" cells. It is very likely that there is a faulty terminal differentiation of T lymphocytes. Our recent studies have shown that levels of terminal deoxynucleotidyl trans-

Table 1. Delayed cutaneous hypersensitivity[3]

Group	Candida	Streptokinase-streptodornase	Trichophyton	DNCB
Healthy (n=50)	36* (7.8±1.9)	37 (15.3±3.6)	27 (6.7±1.8)	50
Protein-energy malnutrition (n=50)	11 (3.9±1.1)	14 (4.1±2.8)	9 (3.3±0.9)	29

* Number showing positive response (induration $\geq$ 5 mm).
  Figures in parentheses refer to the mean ±S.D. diameter of induration for the entire group.

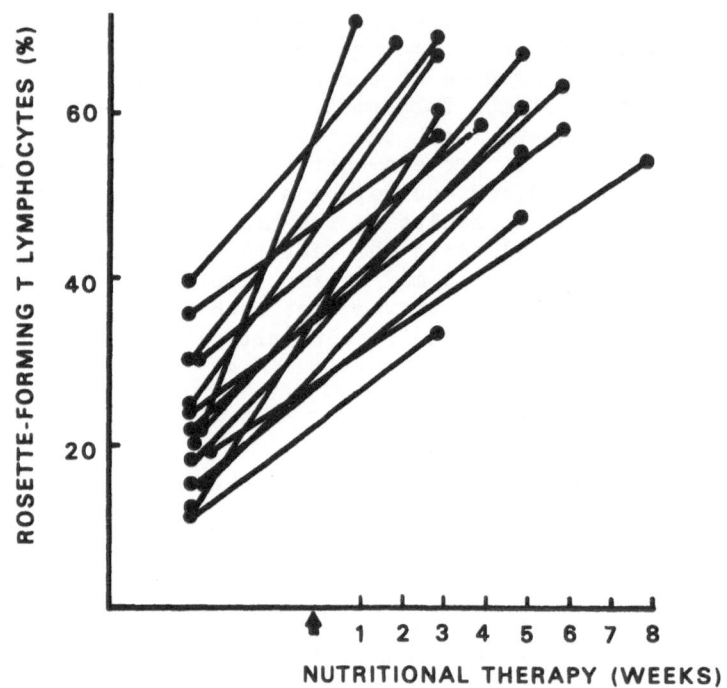

Fig. 2.   Rosette-forming T cells in malnutrition and response to
          therapy[6]

ferase enzyme in leukocytes are increased in malnutrition and these
correlate with the proportion of null cells (Fig. 3)[18]. Furthermore, the addition of thymosin fraction V to mononuclear cell preparations of malnourished individuals results in the increase in
rosetting cells in vitro[19]. The role of impaired thymic inductive
factors is suggested also by reduction in the activity of thymic
hormone in the serum of malnourished children (Fig. 4). Carefully
controlled studies of deprivation in laboratory animals have confirmed that deficiencies of zinc and pyridoxine have an adverse
effect on thymic hormone activity, whereas vitamin A deficiency does
not appear to influence this factor. Finally, cultured thymic epithelium of deprived animals does not induce the differentiation of
stem cells into functionally competent T lymphocytes.

     Intraepithelial lymphocytes have many of the surface character-
istics and functions of effector T lymphocytes. In malnourished
children there was a significant reduction in the number of intraepithelial lymphocytes compared with healthy controls. This is
likely to be the direct result of thymic atrophy associated with

starvation, since neonatal thymectomy in rats produces similar effects and when thymectomised animals are starved the number of intraepithelial lymphocytes is not further reduced. Leakage of these lymphocytes into dilated lymphatics of the villus has also been postulated.

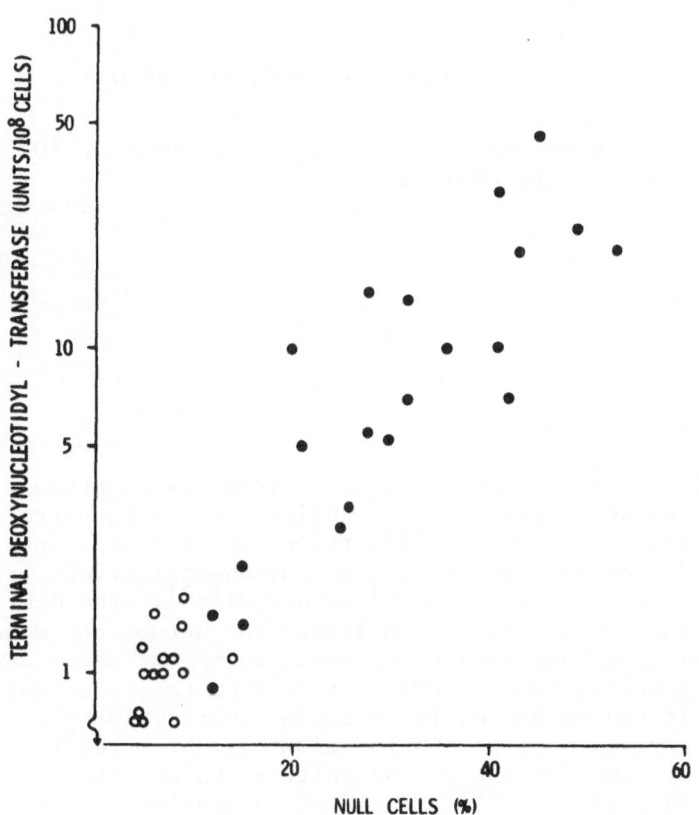

Fig. 3.   Leukocyte TdT levels correlated with the proportion of "null" cells[18]

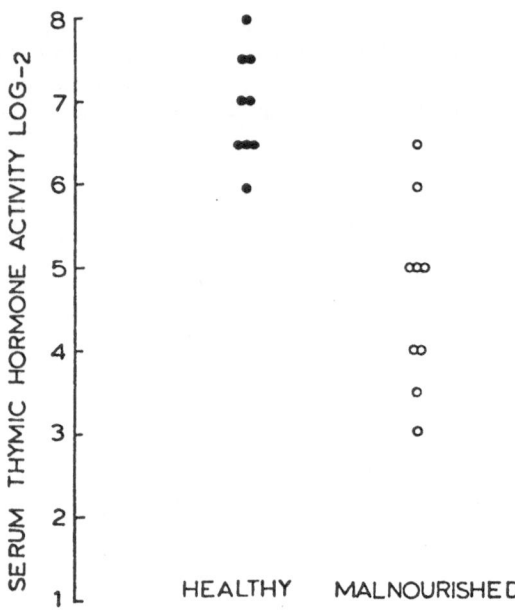

Fig. 4.   Thymic hormone activity in undernourished (O) and
          healthy (●) children.

LYMPHOCYTE PROLIFERATION

     The ability of T lymphocytes to increase DNA synthesis and to
divide in response to mitogens and antigens is an in vitro correlate
of cellular immunity. The proliferative capacity of lymphocytes in
response to polyclonal mitogens, e.g. phytohemagglutinin, has been
variously reported as impaired[20] or normal[21]. The many variables
influencing the final results, including the nature and dose of the
antigen or mitogen, duration of culture, source of serum and number
of responding cells, make an accurate interpretation of data very
difficult. It can be shown, for example, that lymphocyte stimulation
response to phytohaemagglutinin in malnutrition correlates with the
number of rosetting T cells in the culture; those with fewer T
lymphocytes respond less[22]. Serum of malnourished infected
patients inhibits proliferation or fails to support optimal
response[23]. Among other factors, products of microorganisms such

as endotoxin, antigen-antibody complexes, IgE, $alpha_2$ macroglobulin, may influence the results. The absence or reduced concentrations of essential amino acids and trace elements in sera of malnourished children may be important[24].

LYMPHOKINES

There are limited data on the production of lymphokines by sensitised T lymphocytes. Macrophage migration inhibition factor has been found to be somewhat reduced[4], whereas the analogous leukocyte inhibition factor is normally produced in the majority of malnourished children[25]. There is no correlation between the severity of nutritional deficiency and the production of MIF and LIF[26]. The production of interferon has been reported to be reduced in marasmic infants[27] although this may be related to the age of the individual[28].

PRACTICAL SIGNIFICANCE REGARDING IMMUNISATION OF
MALNOURISHED INDIVIDUALS

Since nutritional deficiency is associated with impaired immunological responses, the effectiveness of prophylactic vaccination myst be carefully examined. The extensive literature on antibody production in response to a variety of bacterial, viral, rickettsial and other antigens has been analysed and summarised[6]. It was concluded that the serum antibody level following adequate immunisation is generally normal and that suboptimal response in undernourished subjects can be improved by giving a larger dose of the antigen, choosing appropriate adjuvants, and excluding serious concomitant infection. There have been reports of geographical variations in the response of young children to live attenuated polio virus vaccine. In two studies in India the frequency of seroconversion and titre of antibody were lower, but this was not correlated with nutritional status. Virus "take" indicated by the presence of vaccine virus in the stools was generally associated with positive seroconversion. Antibody response improved and was comparable with titres achieved in trials in industrialised countries when polio virus vaccine was administered five times. Occasionally, some malnourished children show a secondary booster response following the apparently primary administration of an antigen, thereby suggesting previous exposure and memory even though antibody was not detected prior to immunisation. There are few available data on the local mucosal antibody response in malnutrition. This has been examined in only one study in which the presence and levels of secretory IgA

antibody to live attenuated measles and polio virus vaccines were
significantly reduced. Clearly, there is a need for further
information in this important area.

There is limited information on specific cell-mediated immunity
following prophylactic immunisation. Following BCG vaccination,
tuberculin conversion is observed less often in malnourished individuals. This impairment can only partly be overcome by testing
with a higher concentration of purified protein derivative. Low-
birth-weight infants who are small-for-gestation also show reduced
tuberculin conversion and decreased lymphokine production.

The critical factor in this area is the correlation between
nutritional status and protective immunity to infection rechallenge,
irrespective of the magnitude of the immune response produced. The
protective titres of specific antibody in man are not well defined
for most infections. It is conceivable that the lower levels of
immune response encountered in nutritional deficiency syndromes may
still be effective in warding off natural disease. Furthermore,
careful studies are required for the incidence, nature, and severity
of complications in immunised malnourished children following exposure
to natural infection in the community setting. Moreover, most studies
of immunological-nutritional interactions have demonstrated impaired
responses in severe forms of malnutrition, such as kwashiorkor and
marasmus, whereas these patients constitute only 1% to 2% of the malnourished population. The responses to immunisation of individuals
with mild-to-moderate PEM and of those with deficiencies of individual
nutrients should be evaluated. Based on current information, there
is full justification for continuing comprehensive immunisation
programmes in all populations, perhaps with some additional pre-
cautions to ensure an adequate response.

APPLICATION OF AVAILABLE DATA TO PLANNED INTERVENTIONS

Based on information already available, we must consider practical intervention strategies to tackle the widespread problems of
malnutrition and infection. A multifaceted attack on the twin
problems of nutritional deficiency and infection must be mounted.
Human milk contains a number of physiochemical and cellular protective
factors, including lactoferrin, antibodies, phagocytes, and macrophages. Breast feeding is associated with a lower frequency of
diarrhoea and respiratory infections, and complications such as
dehydration and septicaemia also occur less often. These effects
are achieved in all communities but are greatest and most useful in
communities with heavy environmental contamination and poor standards
of personal hygiene. Schedules of vaccination should be improved
to make them more effective. This may necessitate modification with
regard to the amount of antigen, number of inoculations, timing in
respect of of nutritional status, and the type of adjuvants employed.

The demonstration of impaired immune responses in malnutrition has led to preliminary attempts at stimulation of the immune system by cell extracts or pharmacological agents. Three studies have evaluated the effect of the administration of <u>transfer factor</u>. Both the protocols and the results differed. In one, no benefits were seen, whereas in the other there was a reduction in the occurrence of diarrhoea but not in that of chest, middle ear, or skin infections. In our controlled study, transfer factor administration was associated with a decrease in the severity of infection and associated complications but not in the frequency of infectious illnesses. <u>Levamisole</u> has been widely used as an anthelminthic and has been demonstrated to stimulate cell-mediated immunity both <u>in vivo</u> and <u>in vitro</u>. Side effects of its use on a short-term basis are rare. The effects of levamisole administration on cellular immunity in malnutrition have been reported. The role of short-term immunopotentiation with one or more agents in severely malnourished children before or during critical periods of stress, such as infection, requires careful evaluation. At the present time, this must remain an experimental tool with limited practical value.

The provision of nutritional supplements shortly before or during a period of metabolic stress, such as infection, may reduce the impairment of immunity associated with undernutrition. This may be particularly relevant for hospitalised patients. Specific nutrients may be required in individual subjects.

Low birth weight is associated with significant and prolonged impairment of cellular immunity, particularly in those who continue to have physical growth retardation (vide infra). Impaired immunocompetence associated with foetal malnutrition can to some extent be prevented by appropriate antenatal and perinatal practices. The strategies for dealing with this problem must necessarily take into account the prevalence of various risk factors in the community and the magnitude of risk associated with each of these factors.

RECOVERY OF IMMUNOLOGICAL FUNCTION

Nutritional supplementation and clinical improvement are associated with rapid recovery of immune responsiveness. In fact, increase in the number of T lymphocytes may be observed well before clinical and biochemical recovery and this index may provide a good test of therapeutic efficiency (Fig. 2). The exception to this is the small-for-gestation infant who shows persistence of impaired cell-mediated immunity for several months and perhaps years (Fig. 5). (Fig. 5)[29,30,31]. The heterogeneity of causation of fetal growth retardation is recognised and it would be imperative to study the effects of individual causal factors on immunocompetence of the neonate. In laboratory animals deprived of various nutrients,

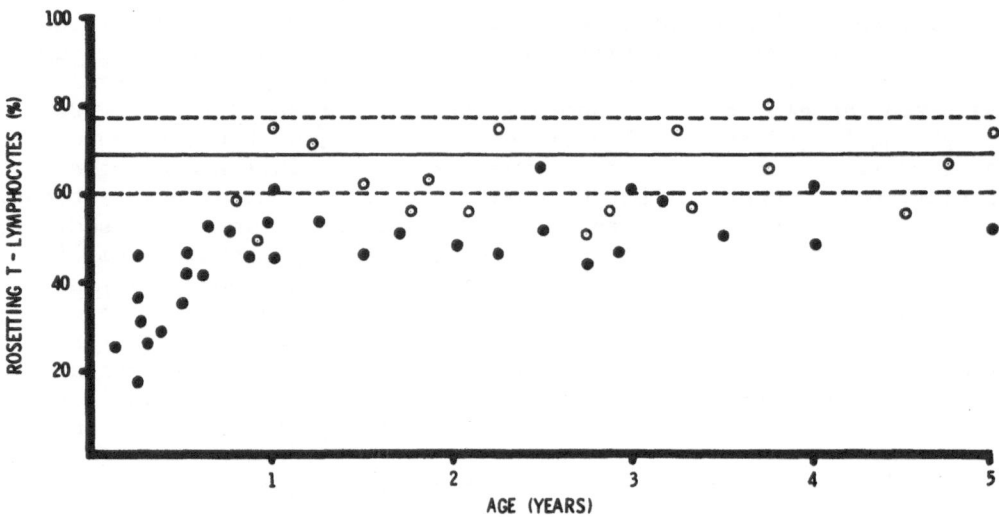

Fig. 5. Rosetting T-cells in low-birth-weight small-for-gestation
         infants with persistent growth retardation (O) and those
         who had had catch up growth (●)

impaired immune response to T-cell dependent antigen is observed in
the offspring even though food is offered ad libitum[32]. The clinical and biological significance of these prenatal influences is not
clear but serious infections including pneumonia and septicaemia are
more common in such growth-retarded infants.

CONCLUDING COMMENTS

     Protein-energy malnutrition results in marked discernible
alteration in host resistance which may explain in part the enhanced
vulnerability of undernourished individuals to infection. However,
we must interpret such observations with a certain degree of caution.
Some of the important considerations in the complex interactions of
nutrition, immunity and infection have been reviewed elsewhere[4].
Malnutrition in man is a complex mixture of deficiency of several
nutrients and various permutations of deficiency syndromes may
produce variable effects of immunocompetence. The techniques of
measuring immunity have serious limitations in terms of sensitivity,
specificity and scatter. One must be careful in extrapolating from
in vitro data to in vivo significance and from information gathered
in laboratory animals to the situation in man. The threshold of
quantitatively significant immunodeficiency needs definition. The
separate effects of malnutrition and infection on immune responses
should be disected carefully.

One hopes that not only would answers be sought to the questions raised above but that the existing knowledge would be used to plan intervention schemes to alleviate the human suffering consequent upon malnutrition and infection.

REFERENCES

1. AMA Expert Panel (1980) J. Amer. Med. Assoc. (in press).
2. Chandra R.K. (1979) Bull. WHO 57: 167.
3. Chandra R.K. (1980) "Immunology of Nutritional Disorders", Edward Arnold, London.
4. Chandra R.K. (1981) in "Immunodeficiency Disorders" ed. Chandra R.K., Churchill Livingstone, Edinburgh.
5. Chandra R.K. (1981) Brit. Med. Bull. 37 (in press).
6. Chandra R.K. and Newberne P.M. (1977) "Nutrition, Immunity and Infection: Mechanisms of Interactions", Plenum, New York.
7. Kahan B.D. (1980) J. Ent. Parent. Nutr. (in press).
8. Scrimshaw N.S., Taylor C.E. and Gordon J.E. (1968) WHO Monograph Series 57.
9. Suskind R.M. (ed.) (1977) "Malnutrition and the Immune Response", Raven Press, New York.
10. Watson R.R. and McMurray D.N. (1979) Crit. Rev. Food. Sci. Nutr. 12: 113.
11. Chandra R.K. (1972) J. Pediatr. 81: 1194.
12. Ziegler H.D. and Ziegler P.B. (1975) John Hopkins Med. J. 137: 59.
13. Abbassy A.S., El-Din M.K., Hassan A.I. et al. (1974) J. Trop. Med. Hyg. 77: 13.
14. Edelman R., Suskind R., Olson R.E. and Sirisinha S. (1973) Lancet i: 506.
15. Kielman A.A., Uberoi I.S., Chandra R.K. and Mehra V.L. (1976) Bull. WHO 54 477.
16. Chandra R.K. (1974) BMJ 3: 608.
17. Chandra R.K. (1977) Pediatrics. 59: 423.
18. Chandra R.K. (1979) Acta Paediat. Scand. 68: 841.
19. Jackson T.M. and Zaman S.N. (1980) Clin. Exp. Immunol. 39: 717.
20. Smythe P.M., Brerton-Stiles G.G., Grace H.J. et al. (1971) Lancet ii: 939.
21. Schlesinger L. and Stekel A. (1974) Am. J. Clin. Nutr. 27: 615.
22. Chandra R.K. (1980) Fed. Proceed. (in press).
23. Moore D.L., Heyworth B. and Brown J. (1977) Immunology 33: 777.
24. Beatty D.W. and Dowdle E.B. (1979) Clin. Exp. Immunol. 35: 433.
25. Heresi G. (1978) Thesis, Universidad de Chile, Santiago, Chile.
26. Lomnitzer R., Rosen E.U., Geefhuysen J. and Rabson A.R. (1976) S. Afr. Med. J. 50: 1820.
27. Schlesinger L., Ohlbaum A., Grez L. and Stekel A. (1976) Am. J. Clin. Nutr. 29: 615.
28. Nichols K. (1980) personal communication.
29. Chandra R.K. (1975) Am. J. Dis. Child. 129: 450.

30.   Chandra R.K. and Bhujwala R.A. (1977) Int. Arch. Allergy Appl.
          Immunol. 53: 180.
31.   Ferguson A.C. (1978) J. Pediat. 93: 51.
32.   Chandra R.K. (1975) Science 190: 289.

ANTIBODY AFFINITY: ITS RELATIONSHIP TO IMMUNE

COMPLEX DISEASE AND THE EFFECT OF MALNUTRITION

M.W. Steward, Madeleine E. Devey, and M.C. Reinhardt[*]

London School of Hygiene and
Tropical Medicine

and

[*]Institute of Child Health
London

INTRODUCTION

There is an impressive body of evidence in the literature to support the view that malnutrition is a major cause of secondary immunodeficiency in man. The malnourished state leads to impaired cell-mediated and humoral immune mechanisms with a consequent predisposition of affected individuals to severe infections. Serum immunoglobulin levels in malnourished individuals are not related to the degree of nutritional impairment and these levels can be high or normal[1]. However, it is clear that specific antibody responses in malnutrition can be adequate or reduced[2]. Whilst it is clear that the amount of antibody an individual makes is important, perhaps more critical to the function of the antibody response is its quality. Antibody affinity is one of the means of expressing antibody quality and is a measure of the strength of interaction of the antibody combining sites with the corresponding antigenic determinants. A high affinity antibody forms complexes with the antigen which have a lesser tendency to dissociate than do complexes formed with a low affinity antibody. In terms of antibody function, high affinity antibody is superior to lower affinity antibody in a number of antibody-mediated immune functions. These include complement fixation, immune elimination, and protective capacity against bacterial infection. Therefore circumstances which interfere with the production of antibody of an appropriate high affinity will result in impaired immune function. The production of antibody of low affinity may be viewed as a form of immunodeficiency[3] leading to the failure of elimination of antigen or infectious agent with the corresponding persistence of infection or the production and subsequent tissue deposition of antigen excess antigen: antibody complexes. The purpose of this paper is to discuss the production of low affinity antibody as an example of a primary immunodeficiency which may predispose to the induction of chronic disease, and to consider how secondary immunodeficiency arising from malnutrition may contribute to disease susceptibility through its effect on antibody affinity.

THE ROLE OF ANTIBODY AFFINITY IN CHRONIC ANTIGEN-ANTIBODY COMPLEX DISEASE

It has been appreciated for many years that the repeated injection of small amounts of foreign serum protein into previously sensitised rabbits results in a chronic glomerulonephritis[4]. These pioneering studies have been extended by workers in many laboratories and a clear relationship has been shown between the presence of circulating antigen-antibody complexes and the development of nephritis[5,6]. The importance of the relative amounts of antibody in the development of disease was suggested and subsequent work by a number of groups[7,8] has shown the importance of the quality of the antibody in soluble complex formation. The proportion of rabbits developing chronic disease (approximately 20%) were those which had non-precipitating (? low avidity) circulating antigen to the injected antigen. Rabbits not developing the disease had precipitating antibody. In an important extension of these studies on the mechanisms underlying chronic immune complex disease, inbred mice were shown to differ in their susceptibility to LCM virus-induced chronic disease; strains which developed the disease failed to eliminate the virus whereas those not developing the disease eliminated the virus efficiently[9]. The presence of circulating complexes of virus and antibody and the renal localisation of these complexes was convincingly demonstrated, showing that the disease was mediated by antigen-antibody complexes and that there were genetically controlled differences in susceptibility. Similar strain-related differences in the development of nephrotic syndrome following infection with Trypanosoma brucei have been demonstrated[10].

It has been argued[3] on both clinical and immunological grounds that susceptibility to chronic antigen-antibody complex disease should be viewed as arising from genetically-controlled immunodeficiency. Based on observations that immunodeficiency is broadly antigen-non-specific and that individuals can produce functionally poor antibodies[11], and considering the work in rabbits and mice described above, it was proposed[3] that chronic antigen-antibody complex disease arises as a result of a genetically-controlled low affinity antibody response. This antibody response fails to eliminate antigen and favours the production, persistence in the circulation and subsequent tissue localisation of antigen-excess complexes.

In support of this hypothesis, it was shown that strains of mice susceptible to chronic disease following LCM virus infection (BIO D2 new and SWR/J) produced lower affinity antibody to a number of antigens injected in saline than did mice not susceptible to chronic disease (C3H, A/JAX)[3,12]. Furthermore, the low affinity antibody producing strains were poorer at active immune elimination of antigen, and passive-transfer of antibody of defined affinity confirmed that low affinity antibody was indeed poorer than high affinity antibody at immune elimination of antigen[13].

The genetic control of antibody affinity to antigens injected in saline implied by these experiments in inbred mice was confirmed by extensive breeding studies[14,15]. These breeding experiments also demonstrated that the genetic control of affinity was independent of those genetic mechanisms controlling antibody levels and was also independent of the antigens of the major histocompatibility complex[16].

The question arises as to the level at which the genetic control of antibody affinity is expressed and a number of possibilities have been discussed: the macrophage[17,18], the T helper cell[19,3] or the B cell[20]. Macrophage function has been studied in detail and when assessed by either carbon clearance or clearance of polyvinyl pyrrolidone (PVP) it differs in inbred strains of mice. A low affinity antibody response to protein antigens is associated with either poor clearance of carbon or a slow recovery of macrophages from blockade by carbon[17] and it is also associated with a poor clearance of ^{125}-I-labelled PVP[18]. Furthermore, carbon blockage reduces the affinity of antibody produced in mice which normally produce high affinity antibody and stilboestrol treatment enhances both macrophage clearance of carbon and antibody affinity. These results suggest a central role for macrophage function in determining the function of high antibody affinity perhaps via appropriate antigen handling and presentation to immunocompetent cells. However, following an extensive breeding programme in which mice were bred according to their ability to produce either high or low affinity antibody to protein antigens, two lines of mice have been generated. One line produces high affinity antibody and the second, low affinity antibody[15]. When macrophage clearance function was measured by PVP clearance, clearance of aggregated IgG and clearance of preformed antigen-antibody complexes, no differences between the two lines were found[21]. These results suggest that in these mice at least, affinity control is exerted at a level other than that measured by clearance function tests and it may be that other factors controlling affinity have been selected in this breeding programme.

THE EFFECTS OF MALNUTRITION

Dietary manipulation of experimental mice has a profound effect upon macrophage clearance function. Animals fed isocaloric diets in which the protein content was restricted to 4% had an impaired clearance of ^{125}-I-PVP (KPVP) compared to those mice receiving normal amounts of protein[22]. This effect could be reversed within three days. In addition, mice receiving diets in which phenylalanine and tryptophan were restricted showed a marked increase in impairment of PVP clearance with decreased amounts of these amino acids[23]. The α_{PVP} increased in both experiments. K_{PVP} presumably reflects the overall phagocytic capacity of the animal and α_{PVP} reflects the activity of individual macrophages.

When mice which normally produce high affinity antibody are subjected to protein malnutrition, macrophage clearance of carbon and antibody affinity are depressed[21]. In low affinity mice macrophage clearance of PVP was decreased on low protein diets but antibody affinity was not reduced. It seems likely, therefore, that malnutrition could lead to impaired macrophage function, a low affinity antibody response, the failure to eliminate infectious agents and the production, persistence and deposition of injurious antigen-antibody complexes.

THE INDUCTION OF CHRONIC ANTIGEN-ANTIBODY COMPLEX DISEASE
IN LOW AND HIGH AFFINITY MICE

Preliminary experiments on the induction of chronic antigen-antibody complex disease in inbred mice by repeated injections of protein antigens were performed in high affinity and low affinity mice. After six weeks of repeated injection of human serum albumin, the low affinity SWR/J mice had higher levels of circulating HSA-anti-HSA complexes in the circulation than did the high affinity Simpson mice. Furthermore, SWR/J mice showed a significantly reduced glomerular filtration rate compared to Simpson mice and uninjected controls[24].

The availability of high and low affinity lines of mice produced from the same parent population by a process of selective breeding, based on the affinity of antibody to protein antigens injected in saline, afforded an ideal opportunity to assess the relationship of antibody affinity to the development of chronic antigen-antibody complex disease. Accordingly, mice were injected daily with human serum albumin and glomerular filtration rate, proteinuria, levels of circulating complexes and the localisation of complexes in the glomeruli by immunofluorescence were assessed. The results obtained demonstrated that mice selected to produce a lower average affinity response to protein antigens develop more severe chronic disease than mice selected for higher affinity antibody production. The low

affinity mice had (a) higher levels of circulating antigen-antibody
complexes; (b) a greater impairment of renal function; (c) greater
proteinuria; (d) a greater deposition of complexes in the glomeruli;
(e) a greater incidence of glomerular basement membrane localisation
of complexes and (f) a greater number of deaths from renal failure
than high affinity mice[25,26]. In high affinity mice, where complexes were localised in the glomeruli, they were seen in the mesangium rather than on the basement membrane as in the low affinity
mice.

These results show that the characteristic of low affinity
antibody production is indeed associated with the development of
severe complex-induced glomerulonephritis. Work from other laboratories is consistent with this view. Following prolonged immunisation
of rabbits with ovalbumin, the production of low avidity, non-
precipitating antibody was associated with diffuse membrano-
proliferative glomerulonephritis whereas mesangio-proliferative
nephritis was associated with the production of high avidity precipitating antibodies[8].

In passive acute nephritis in mice, complexes composed of high
affinity rabbit anti-DNP antibodies were localised in the mesangium
whereas those composed of low affinity anti-DNP were localised on
the basement membrane[27]. In a similar system, low affinity rabbit
antibodies gave rise to diffuse proliferative glomerulonephritis
with sub-epithelial deposits[28].

THE EFFECT OF MALNUTRITION ON ANTIGEN-ANTIBODY COMPLEX DISEASE

F_1 hybrid mice of the NZB and NZW strains (NZB/W F_1) have been
extensively studied because they develop a disease which closely
resembles human systemic lupus erythematosus. The animals develop
various T-cell deficiencies, antibodies to ds DNA and later to
erythrocytes. They also develop increasing levels of circulating
complexes with increasing age[29,30] and an immune complex glomerulonephritis in which complexes of ds DNA-anti-DNA, ss DNA-anti-ss DNA
and virus antigen-antivirus antibody complexes are deposited in the
kidneys[31]. Dietary manipulation has been shown to have pronounced
effects upon the development of autoimmune disease in the NZB
mice[32,33,34]. Diets high in fat and low in protein and fibre
accelerated the development of autoimmunity and shortened life whereas low fat high protein, high fibre diets delayed autoimmunity and
increased life. Protein restriction but normal caloric intake
delayed the loss of T-cell functions. The immune complex disease
of the NZB/W F_1 mice is also markedly affected by dietary manipulation. The lifespan of NZB/W mice is prolonged by restriction of
caloric intake[35] and the restriction of the intake of phenylamine
and tyrosine prolonged the life of the F_1 hybrids and prevented the
development of renal disease[36]. Restriction of diets of NZB/W
mice to 10 kcal per day from the time of weaning resulted in reduced

levels of antibodies to ds DNA, an inhibition of the deposition of
immunoglobulin in the gomerular capillaries[37] and a significant
reduction in the levels of circulating antigen-antibody complexes[38].
Furthermore, over 95% of NZB/W mice fed diets rich in saturated or
unsaturated fats developed severe immune complex disease and died
sooner than littermate controls fed a low fat diet[39]. It is clear
from this work that malnutrition of these mice results in an impairment of the development of their autoimmune and immune-complex
diseases. We have investigated the effect of protein restriction on
the development of chronic renal disease in genetically-selected
high and low affinity mice[40]. Mice of both high and low affinity
lines were fed diets of either 15% or 4% protein and half were
injected daily with 0.25 mg HSA. During the course of the experiment,
glomerular filtration rate was assessed by measurement of the clearance of ^{51}Cr-EDTA. Circulating antigen-antibody complexes were
detected by the solid-phase C1q and conglutinin binding assays.
Glomerular localisation of complexes in cryostat sections was
assessed by immunofluorescence (Table 1).

Mice receiving the 15% diet responded to the daily injections
of HSA as previously described[24,26]. Low affinity mice had more
severe renal impairment (50% had died by the seventieth injection),
a greater localisation of complexes involving capillary loops and
higher levels of circulating complexes, detected by both methods,
than did high affinity mice. Mice receiving 4% diet all showed a
decreased glomerular filtration rate compared to normally-fed
controls. Low affinity mice receiving 4% diet and daily injections
of albumin again had a greater renal impairment and a greater incidence of complex deposition in the capillary loops compared to high
affinity mice. The intensity of complex deposition although still
greater in the low affinity mice was lower than in mice receiving
15% diet. There were no deaths in either group. Levels of circulating complexes detected by both methods in the low affinity mice
receiving the 4% diet were reduced but levels detected by the C1qBA
were increased. No complexes were detected in the high affinity
mice by either assay. Free antibody in the circulation of both
lines of mice 24 hours after the last antigen injection was significantly reduced in mice receiving the 4% diet, but were not different
between the two lines. Antibody affinity was, however, low in both
lines on both 15% and 4% diets. The failure to detect high affinity
antibody in the serum of high affinity line mice may have arisen
from the binding of high affinity antibody to the infected antigen,
followed by the clearance of antigen-antibody complexes containing
this high affinity antibody and a corresponding reduction in the
average affinity value measured. Although protein deprivation is
known to reduce antibody affinity in high affinity line mice[21],
it did not result in an increased incidence of chronic disease in
these mice injected daily with HSA. This may have arisen as a
result of immunosuppression of overall antibody levels to a level
insufficient to cause immune complex deposition. Alternatively, the

Table 1.   The effect of protein deprivation on chronic antigen-antibody complex disease in genetically selected mice

	15% protein diet		4% protein diet	
	Low affinity mice	High affinity mice	Low affinity mice	High affinity mice
GFR	very reduced	normal	reduced	normal
Immunofluorescence				
% positive: anti-Ig	100	40	54	45
anti-C3	63	0	27	0
anti-HSA	88	10	54	18
Predominant localisation of complexes	mesangiocappillary + capillary	mesangiocappillary + mesangial	mesangiocappillary + capillary	mesangiocapillary + mesangial
Circulating complexes				
KBA	+++	-	-	+
ClqBA	++	-	+++	-
Free antibody after 73 injections:				
Levels (Abt, p moles/10ul)	924 577	313 274	400 301	227 + 151
Affinity (x 10 L/M)	0.40 0.21	0.34 0.25	0.21 0.08	0.27 0.10

immunoglobulin class or subclass of the antibody may not have been appropriate for deposition in the glomeruli. It is also possible that the genetic selection procedure we used which selects for either low affinity or high affinity antibody may also select for properties which affect the susceptibility of the kidney to complex deposition i.e. mesangial function, monocyte infiltration, haemodynamic factors and capillary permeability. According to this view, high affinity mice although producing low affinity antibody as a result of the dietary manipulation, would not develop severe chronic renal disease because of the inherent properties of their kidneys.

The reduction in severity of chronic antigen–antibody complex disease we observed in low affinity mice fed a protein restricted diet is in accordance with the data of Fernandes and his colleagues as described above. This reduction may have arisen as a result of the depression of antibody levels or an alteration in the immuno-globulin class or subclass of the antibody produced. If, as we have suggested[24,25] it is that proportion of high affinity antibody even in a low average affinity antibody population which is actually deposited in the glomeruli then protein deprivation may have elimi-nated this small population of antibodies from low affinity mice. Thus the severity of their disease would be reduced.

Levels of circulating complexes in low affinity mice detected by the KBA were very reduced on protein deptrivation. However, complexes detected by the ClqBa were raised in these mice. We have demonstrated that the KBA detects smaller complexes than does the ClqBa[26] and the reduced severity of the chronic disease in low affinity mice may have arisen as a result of the production of these larger complexes which would tend to localise in the mesangium rather than on the basement membrane[28]. This explanation is not totally consistent with the above suggestion of the elimination of the high affinity subpopulation in protein-restricted low affinity mice because it may be expected that large complexes would be composed of high affinity antibody. The reduction in the levels of circulating complexes in NZB/W mice was achieved by feeding low caloric diets but our diets were isocaloric[38]. Thus the mechanisms by which immune complex levels are influenced are clearly complicated.

Whatever the mechanisms involved, dietary manipulation of our low affinity mice does reduce the severity of chronic antigen–antibody complex disease. Whether the site of modification is primarily immunological or whether protein restriction affects renal functions such as mesangial uptake or capillary permeability etc. remains to be investigated.

CONCLUSION

Malnutrition exerts a profound immunosuppressive effect upon humoral antibody responses. The mechanisms by which these effects are induced are not fully understood but may include effects upon macrophages. The possibility exists that dietary insufficiencies may result in impaired immune responses, including the synthesis of poor quality antibody, which may in turn lead to poor elimination of infective agents and the production of tissue-damaging antigen-excess complexes. The renal disease thus induced may then result in protein loss and further immunosuppression.

ACKNOWLEDGEMENTS

The authors acknowledge the financial support of the Wellcome Trust for part of their work described here. MCR was supported by a fellowship of the Royal Society in its European eschange programme with the Swiss Foundation for Scientific Research.

REFERENCES

1. McFarlane H. (1973) Adv. Clin Chem. 16; 154.
2. Chandra R.K. and Newberne P.M. (1977) "Nutrition, Immunity and Infection", Plenum Press, New York.
3. Soothill J.F. and Steward M.W. (1971) Clin. Exp. Immunol. 9: 193.
4. Longcope W.T. (1913) J. Exp. Med. 18: 678.
5. Germuth F.G. and Rodriguez E. (1971) "Immunopathology of the Renal Glomerulus", Little, Brown & Co., Boston.
6. Dixon F.J., Feldman J.D. and Vasquez J.J. (1961) J. Exp. Med. 113: 899.
7. Pincus T., Haberkern R. and Christian C.L. (1968) J. Exp. Med. 28: 224.
8. Kuriyama T. (1973) Lab. Invest. 28: 224.
9. Oldstone M.B.A. and Dixon F.J. (1969) J. Exp. Med. 129: 583.
10. Soothill J.F., Smith M.D. and Morgan A.G. (1975) in "Pathalogic Processes in Parasitic Infections", Taylor A.E.R. and Muller R. eds., Blackwell, Oxford.
11. Blecher T.E., Soothill J.F., Voyce M.A. and Walker W.H.C. (1968) Clin. Exp. Imm. 3: 47.
12. Petty R.E., Steward M.W. and Soothill J.F. (1972) Clin. Exp. Imm. 12: 231.
13. Alpers J.H., Steward M.W. and Soothill J.F. (1972) Clin. Exp. Imm. 12: 121.
14. Steward M.W. and Petty R.E. (1976) Immunol. 22: 47.
15. Katz F.E. and Steward M.W. (1975) Immunol. 29: 543.
16. Steward M.W., Reinhardt M.C. and Staines N.A. (1979) Immunol. 37: 697.

17. Passwell J.M., Steward M.W. and Soothill J.F. (1974) Clin.
       Exp. Imm. 19: 159.
18. Morgan A.G. and Soothill J.F. (1975) Nature 254: 711.
19. Gershon R.K. and Paul W.E. (1971) J. Immunol. 106: 872.
20. Steward M.W., Gaze S.E. and Petty R.E. (1974) Eur. J. Imm. 4:
       751.
21. Reinhardt M.C. and Steward M.W. (1979) Immunol. 38: 735.
22. Coovadia H.M. and Soothill J.F. (1976) Clin. Exp. Imm. 23: 373.
23. Coovadia H.M. and Soothill J.F. (1976) Clin. Exp. Imm. 23: 562.
24. Steward M.W. (1979) J. Clin. Path. (Suppl. Roy. Coll. Path)
       13: 120.
25. Steward M.W. (1979) Clin. Exp. Imm. 38: 414.
26. Devey M.E. and Steward M.W. (1980) Immunol. (in press).
27. Koyama A., Niwa Y., Shigematsu H., Taniguchi M. and Tada T.
       (1976) Lab. Invest. 35: 293.
28. Germuth F.G., Rodriguez E., Lovelle C.A., Trump E.I., Milano L.
       and Wise O'L (1979) Lab. Invest. 41: 360.
29. Steward M.W. and Powis P.A. (1977) in "Non-articular Forms of
       Rheumatoid Arthritis", Feltkamp T.E.W. ed., Staflen, Leiden,
       p. 23.
30. Andrews B.S., Eisenburg R.A., Theophilopoulous A.N., Izui S.,
       Wilson C.B., McConacney P.J., Murphey E.D. Roths J.B. and
       Dixon F.J. (1978) J. Exp. Med. 148: 1498.
31. Lambert P.H. and Dixon F.J. (1968) J. Exp. Med. 127: 507.
32. Fernandes G., Yunis E.J., Smith J. and Good R.A. (1972) PSEBM
       139: 1189.
33. Fernandes G., Yunis F.J., Jose D.G. and Good R.A. (1973) Int.
       Arch. Allergy Appl. Immunol. 4: 770.
34. Fernandes G., Yunis E.J. and Good R.A. (1976) J. Immunol. 116:
       782.
35. Fernandes G., Yunis E.J. and Good R.A. (1976) Proc. Nat. Acad.
       Sci. 73: 1279.
36. Dubois E.Z. and Strain L. (1973) Biochem. Med. 7: 336.
37. Fernandes G., Friend P., Yunis E.J. and Good R.A. (1978) Proc.
       Nat. Acad. Sci. 75: 1500.
38. Safai Kutti S., Fernandes G., Wang Y., Safai B., Good R.A. and
       Day N.K. (1980) Clin. Immunol. Immunopath. 15: 293.
39. Ibrahim A.B., Gardner M.B. and Levey J.A. (1980) Fed. Proc.
       39: 1132.
40. Reinhardt M.C., Devey M.E., Gregory B., Collins M. and
       Steward M.W. (1980) (in preparation).

IMMUNOLOGICAL IMPLICATIONS OF ALTERNATIVES TO MOTHER'S MILK

I   INFANT FORMULAS

Brian Wharton

Sorrento and Birmingham Maternity Hospitals
Birmingham
United Kingdom

INFANT FORMULAS FOR 'NORMAL' BABIES

Most babies who are not breast fed receive instead a formula based on cow's milk. Without modification cow's milk is unsuitable for infant feeding, mainly because of its high mineral and protein content. Modification of cow's milk for infant feeding is a phenomenon mainly of this century. Continental paediatricians used lactic acid milk partly as an anti-infective measure and partly because the curd tension was reduced. The present generation of infant formulas dates from work initiated by Gerstanberger and Ruh[1,2] in America. Britain was very slow to adopt modified formulas and until the time of the Oppe report "Present Day Practice in Infant Feeding"[3] most British babies received a formula based on whole cow's milk, added vitamins and iron.

Types of formulas

Cow's milk has been modified in three major ways to bring its composition closer to that of breast milk. To understand these modifications various products of the dairy industry (Fig. 1) must be considered -- whole milk, skim milk (a byproduct of butter manufacture), whey (whey protein plus lactose) plus minerals and water -- a byproduct of cheese manufacture), and demineralised whey. THe modifications of cow's milk may be described as "added carbohydrate", "substituted fat", and "demineralised whey" formulas (Fig. 2, Tables 1 and 2).

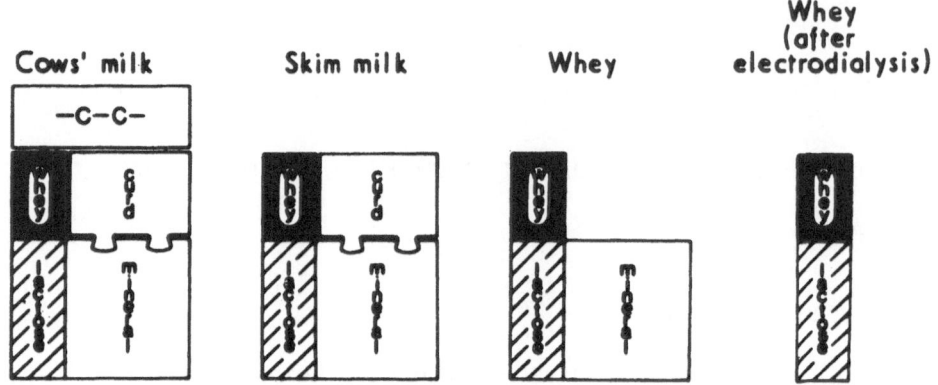

Fig. 1. Products of dairy industry which are used in manufacture of
         infant formulas: whole cow's milk; skim milk (a byproduct
         of butter manufacture); whey, consisting of whey protein,
         lactose, minerals, and water (a byproduct of cheese manu-
         facture) and whey demineralised by electrodialysis.

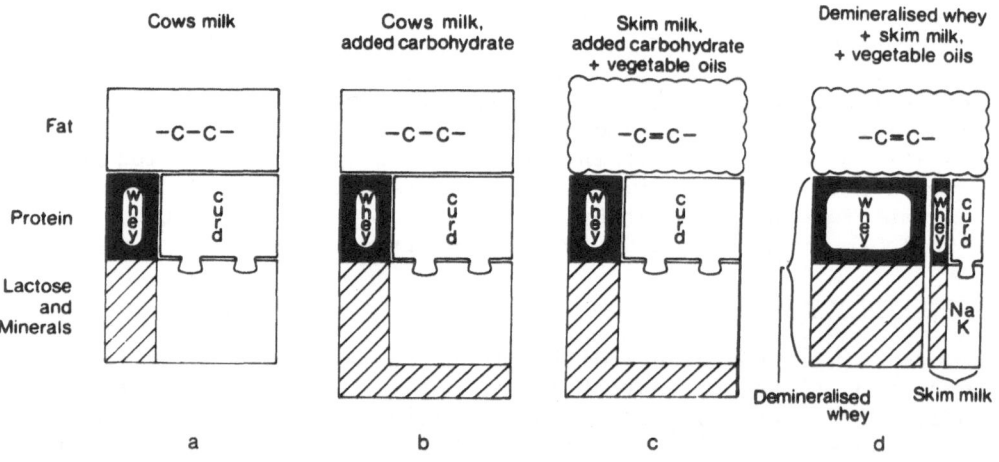

Fig. 2. Modifications of whole cow's milk (a) in manufacture of
        infant formulas; (b) added carbohydrate; (c) substituted
        fat; and (d) demineralised whey.

(From Wharton and Berger[4], by kind permission of ther Editor,
British Medical Journal.)

Table 1. Examples of different types of infant formulas.

Type 1 Added carbohydrate formulas

    Cow and Gate Plus   Ostermilk Complete
                                   (maltodextrin)

                               Vokra D M (maltodextrin)

                               New Improved Ostermilk 2
                                   (maltodextrin)

Type 2 Substituted fat formulas

      Enfalac   Guigolac (maltodextrin)

      Enfamil   Humana baby-fit
                                (sucrose and maltodextrin)

      Multival   Milumil (maltodextrin and
                                 starch)

      Nativa 2

      Similac

      SMA

Type 3 Demineralised whey formulas

      Anfilac   Almiron
                                (sucrose, maltodextrin)

      Cow and Gate Premium   Aptmil (sucrose,
                                maltodextrin and starch)

      Edamater   Babylac (sucrose)

      Frisolac   Masena adaptado
                                (maltodextrin)

      Humana 0, 1

      Laitguigoz /^{er} age

      Nan

      Natival

      Nutrilon

      Osterfeed

      Pre-Amtimil

      SMA Gold Cap - S26

Table 2. Nutrients of possible immunological significance in breast milk, cow's milk and the various types of formulas -- all values per 100 ml.

Milks and Formulas	Protein[a]							Lactose g	Iron µg	Phosphorus mg	Formula used as example
	Total protein g	Casein mg	Total whey protein mg	α Lactalbumin mg	β Lactoglobulin mg	Lactoferrin mg	Immuno-globulin mg				
Breast milk	1.3	500	800	310		150	150	7.4	76	15	
Added lactose	1.8	1400	400	65	160		55	7.1	650	50	Cow & Gate Plus
Added maltodextrin	1.8	1400	400	65	160		55	5.3[b]	890	53	Improved Ostermilk No.2
Substituted fat	1.9	1500	400	70	170		60	6.4[b]	700	55	Milumil
Demineralised whey	1.5	600	900	150	400		125	7.2	1300	33	SMA Gold Cap
Cow's milk	3.4	2700	700	120	300		100[c]	4.8	50	95	

(a)   As nitrogen, i.e. allowance for non-protein nitrogen has not been made.

(b)   Also contains maltodextrin.

(c)   Mainly Ig and Igm, mainly IgA in human milk.

Added carbohydrate formulas. The simplest modification of cow's milk, the addition of carbohydrate, not only increases the overall concentration of carbohydrate but also reduces (dilutes) the concentration of protein, fat and minerals per unit energy intake (Fig. 2b). There are some problems in deciding which carbohydrate to add. Should all of it be lactose, the gut of some babies would be unable to handle this amount, resulting in lactose malabsorption and fermentative diarrhoea. Therefore, instead of adding only lactose, a small amount of fat as well as lactose or a different carbohydrate such as maltodextrins or sucrose may be added.

Substituted fat formulas. The composition of a substituted fat formula -- that is, replacement of the cow's milk fat with a mixture of vegetable and animal fats whose fatty acid compositions more closely approximate to that of breast milk, shown in Fig. 2c. The absorption of fat from such formulas is higher than from cow's milk and approaches that from breast milk.

Demineralised whey formulas. Formulas based on demineralised whey have been used increasingly in recent years (Fig. 2d). Demineralised whey, containing whey protein and a low concentration of minerals, is used as the base and to this is added a small amount of skim milk, so introducing curd protein, further lactose, and some minerals in their naturally occurring form, while other minerals such as copper, iron, zinc, and sometimes manganese may be added individually. A fat mixture and vitamins are added to complete the formula. The protein in the formula is about equal curd and whey as in human milk, while the concentrations of major electrolytes, calcium and phosphorus, are reduced and are much nearer to those of breast milk than can be achieved by adding carbohydrate alone, probably because of the greater cysteine content of whey protein, and there is an advantage for human infants in the early weeks of   life (Tables 1 and 2)

Acid-base properties of the formula

The various modifications of cow's milk described above result in a number of changes in the acid-base properties of the formulas produced, some of which may have microbiological and immunological significance.

Physical chemistry and faecal flora. The preponderance of lactobacilli in the stools of breast fed babies has been explained broadly along the following lines[5]. Not all of the lactose in breast milk is absorbed, indeed normal breast fed babies excrete lactose in their stools. The large bowel, therefore, contains small amounts of lactose which favours the growth of lactobacilli and as acid is generated from the bacterial metabolism of the lactose, the low pH also favours the growth of lactobacilli rather than E. coli. The low phosphate and casein contents of breast milk limit its buffering capacity (buffering capacity can be defined or measured as the amount of hydrochloric acid necessary to reduce the pH to 5), and so this low pH is maintained, again favouring the growth of lactobacilli. In addition there are various acids which with their salts form buffer systems such as bicarbonate and citrate which apart form their buffering properties may affect the intestinal flora via interactions with iron and lactoferrin.

When the added carbohydrate in a type 1 formula is only lactose, this might presumably mimic the higher lactose content of breast milk. Somilarly the reduction in phosphate concentration of all three types of formula, the moderate reduction in casein content of types 1 and 2, and the substantial reduction in type 3, by reducing buffering capacity might again mimic the microbiological properties of breast milk.

In vitro acid base properties. There is not much information about the acid base properties of infant formulas. We have made a number of determinations on representative formulas. Generally the values are between those of breast milk and cow's milk, and the demineralised whey formula had the lowest buffering capacity, presumably reflecting the lower casein and very low phosphate content. Care is necessary in extrapolating from these in vitro observations to the metabolic effects on the babies in vivo. In most milks and formulas the measured titratable acid is mainly citric acid which after absorption is rapidly metabolised to carbon dioxide and so does not contribute to the net load of metabolic acid. The major sources of acid in vivo are from the endogenous production of organic acids, of sulphuric acid from sulphur amino acids, and from hydrogen ions released during bone deposition[6,7]. These strictures do not apply when considering the effect of the formula in the gut although its early intraluminal digestion may well alter its acid-base characteristics and hence its microbiological effect.

Effects of infant formulas on faecal flora. The number of studies is small. When sodium bicarbonate was added to cow's milk to bring its pH to between 7.2 and 7.4 the increased bacteriostatic effect in vitro of the milk reduced the stool pH from 5.9 to 5.5 and led to a change in stool flora so that lactobacilli predominated[8]. In some ways these changes are difficult to interpret in terms of the mechanisms discussed above because the addition of alkali would increase the buffering capacity, at least as measured by titration with hydrochloric acid as indeed we found when sodium and potassium citrate was added to a formula[7]. Similar results were obtained when the pH was raised with trometamole, although this has not been confirmed in other studies[9,10].

I am unaware of any studies of the microbiological effect of adding carbohydrate even though this might be expected to induce changes; the possible differences in the effects of added maltodextrins as opposed to added lactose deserves study. Similarly the effect of substituted fat has not been studied although there seems no reason why this manoeuvre of food technology should have any microbiological sequels unless by chance the fat blend substituted contained the C18:2 fatty acid which occurs in breast milk and has antistaphylococcal activity, at least in mice[11]. The effects of two demineralised whey formulas have been studied and the results compared with the effects of cow's milk and breast milk. The stools of the babies receiving these formulas had a pH of between that seen in babies receiving breast milk or cow's milk, but mostly the stools were more like those of babies fed cow's milk in that clostridia were present in significant numbers, bacteroides counts were mostly higher than in breast-fed babies, after the first week or so coliforms predominated, propionic and volatile fatty acids were usually present while acetate buffer was only occasionally present[9,12]. The stools were so similar to those of babies on unmodified cow's milk that one wonders whether the role of casein, phosphate, and buffering capacity is less important in determining the faecal flora than has been thought.

The same group in Luton studied the effect of a very synthetic formula designed to mimic the microbiological effect of breast milk[13]. The stools of these babies were very similar to those of breast-fed babies: the pH was 5, lactobacilli were found in 53% of the babies compared to 68% of those breast-fed and 39% of those fed cow's milk. Proteus, pseudomonas and clostridia were found in about as many babies as the breast-fed group. The formula was based on whey (not stated to be demineralised), a protein hydrolysate, extra lactose and cream and so probably had a high mineral content (from the whey powder) and a high osmolality and titratable acidity (from the protein hydrolysate). Similarly, the amount of sodium bicarbonate added to cow's milk by Harrison and Peate[7] would lead to an excessive sodium content and renal solute load. Such formulas would not be immediately suitable for widespread use in infant feeding, but the principle seems worthy of further study and development.

It seems then that a lot of information is still needed, e.g. the effects of different carbohydrates. Babies consuming currently available formulas produce stools which are microbiologically very similar to those produced by babies on unmodified cow's milk; experimental formulas can be produced which mimic many of the microbiological effects of breast milk and which may form a basis for future development, but at present they would not be acceptable for general use in early infancy.

Protein properties

Lactoferrin. Cow's milk contains only traces of lactoferrin so that only negligible amounts are found even in formulas based on demineralised whey. Bovine colostrum contains more lactoferrin than mature human milk and genetic selection might result in cows producing significant amounts of lactoferrin throughout their lactation rather than only in colostrum. Bovine colostrum is not inhibitory in vitro at its natural pH because of the high concentration of citrate which competes with lactoferrin for iron and makes it available for bacterial growth[14], and this is true of human milk; the bacteriostatic action of human milk due to the combined action of lactoferrin and antibody depends on the addition of bicarbonate to counteract the iron mobilising effect of citrate[15]. The contents of bicarbonate and citrate in milk and their absorption and secretion in the intestine may, therefore, be very important in the immunological qualities of milk, but they have received little attention; indeed the concentration of these substances in most formulas is not stated. In the absence of lactoferrin, however, their immunological importance may be limited to their contribution to buffering capacity.

Immunoglobulin. Cow's milk contains very little IgA -- about 3% of that in human milk. Attempts have been made, however, to increase its immunoglobulin concentration by immunisation. Pregnant cows were immunised with a polyvalent E. coli vaccine and the whey proteins separated from colostrum collected during the first ten days of lactation. The whey proteins had anti E. coli activity as measured by passive haemagglutination and a mouse protection test.

There were three groups of clinical observations. Infants receiving 2 g per kg per day of the whey proteins had stools containing both intact and fragmented immunoglobulin which conserved their protective activity in mice. In further studies in Barcelona and Lille 156 children with E. coli gastroenteritis received whey proteins. E. coli disappeared from the stools of over half of the treated children compared to about a third of the controls[16].

Clearly much more work is necessary before these observations can be translated into infant feeding practice, but they are promising.

Allergenicity of protein. Presumably any of the individual proteins in cow's milk may induce specific antibody and provoke allergy in a susceptible child, but some proteins seem more antigenic than others.

(a) Antigenicity of different proteins. Animal experiments suggest that β lactoglobulin is more antigenic than either casein or the small amount of α lactalbumin found in cow's milk[17]. Compiled data from five studies of cow's milk protein intolerance in infancy showed sensitivity to β lactoglobulin in 82%, casein in 43%, α lactalbumin in 41%, bovine serum globulin in 27%, bovine serum albumin in 18%[18].

The use of demineralised whey formulas may, therefore, increase the intake of potential antigen. In practice this does not have any obvious ill effect. Demineralised whey formulas have been increasingly used in recent years in Britain without any obvious increase in the prevalence of cow's milk protein intolerance. However, clinical epidemiology is always difficult even when a condition is easily defined, but the criteria of diagnosis for milk protein intolerance are far from uniform.

Animal and in vitro observations support this clinical evidence. In a series of experiments in Cambridge, the cow's milk protein sensitivity of guinea-pigs drinking different preparations of cow's milk and infant formulas was determined by the incidence of passive cutaneous anaphylaxis and the occurrence of generalised anaphylaxis following intravenous challenge with β lactoglobulin or casein. Generally anaphylactic sensitivity to β lactoglobulin was less common and less severe than to casein. A demineralised whey formula which contained relatively large amounts of β lactoglobulin caused less sensitivity to both β lactoglobulin and casein than a substituted fat formula which contained mainly casein, and a liquid concentrate of the demineralised whey formula caused even less sensitivity[19].

(b) Effect of heat treatment. These observations can be added to those of Sperstein et al[20] who used in vitro precipitation and passive cutaneous anaphylaxis, and found that the antigenicity of casein β lactoglobulin and α lactalbumin was considerably reduced by current commercial milk processing. Evaporation has more effect than spray drying, and drying more effect than pasteurisation[19,20]. These differential observations presumably reflect the effect of heat in reducing the potential allergenicity of β lactoglobulin more than that of casein. Heat processing causes a number of changes in milk including the breakage of disulphide bonds. Casein is relatively heat stable up to boiling point. β lactoglobulin has intermediate heat stability while α lactalbumin is very heat labile; its antigenicity is altered by pasteurisation and almost completely destroyed by procedures used in preparation of infant formulas[22,23].

Nevertheless an overall critical evaluation is difficult; with our presently variable criteria the epidemiology is necessarily weak; are the in vitro and animal observations necessarily of clinical significance? Infant feeding policies are usually based on observations in groups of children, i.e. one is looking for uniformity, not the idiosyncratic[24]. This approach may be incorrect when considering immunological implications when a significant minority of children may have genetically induced immunological traits which make them abnormally sensitive to potential environmental allergens.

It could be that the reduction in allergenicity following heat treatment is insufficient to prevent allergic disease in the genetically
susceptible while the reduction is of little importance to those who
are not susceptible.

(c) Cot death. The problem if individuality is illustrated by
the enigma of cot death; some immunologists have implicated immunological processes in its aetiology[25], but others doubt it[26,27].

(d) Immunological tolerance. Probably many babies are tolerant
of the foreign immunological environment of cow's milk protein. In
one study cow's milk specific IgE was found only in breast-fed babies
and was not present in 54 bottle-fed babies. It was suggested that
the breast-fed babies had received small amounts of cow's milk formula
and became sensitised to it, whereas those who were fed entirely on
cow's milk had been inhibited by the very large amount of allergen
received[28]. Tolerance to cow's milk protein has been observed in
guinea-pigs if they receive the protein in the first two days of
life[29].

To summarise, the potential allergenicity of cow's milk protein,
as indicated by in vitro and animal observations, is reduced by the
processes used in the manufacture of infant formulas. It is uncertain whether this reduction is on the one hand of value to the
majority of infants or on the other hand sufficient for the minority
with genetic susceptibility.

Iron

All cow milk infant formulas contain added iron, mostly at
approximately 10 mg per litre although a few manufacturers produce
formulas with substantially less. This practice meets the
recommendation of the Committee on Nutrition of the American Academy
of Paediatrics concerning iron supplementation for infants[30].
Iron deficiency is still a major problem of infancy even in developed
countries[31], and fortification of infant formulas and other foods,
such as cereals, is an accepted method of dealing with the problem.
Fortified baby foods and cereals provide half of the total iron
intake of children aged six to eighteen months in Britain[32]. Iron
is less well absorbed from infant formulas than from breast milk and
may be as low as 4% of intake[33].

Nevertheless, it is well-known that the bacteriostatic effects
of serum and milk can be abolshed by addition of iron which satu-
rates the iron-binding proteins and provides free iron for bacterial
multiplication[34,35]. Compared to the adult, plasma transferrin
in the newborn is at lower concentration and is more saturated with
iron[36]. There is some clinical evidence that parenteral iron given
to newborn Maori children in an attempt to prevent iron deficiency

in later infancy, resulted in an excessive prevalence of meningitis and septicaemia, presumably due to saturation of the plasma transferrin[37].

Is it justified, therefore, to fortify infant formulas with iron? The present infant formulas do not contain iron binding proteins in any concentration and so there is no antibacterial system which can be ruined by iron. Cow's milk formulas without added iron have little inhibitory effect in vitro on the multiplication of E. coli[38]. Since formulas fortified with iron lead to only a modest increase in plasma transferrin saturation[39,40] it is similarly unlikely that their use would substantially reduce the bacteriostatic activity of the infants plasma -- but I am unaware of a specific study of plasma bacteriostatic activity in breast-fed babies receiving an iron fortified formula. Certainly epidemiological studies have not shown that iron fortification leads to increased morbidity and some have shown a reduction in the prevalence of infection[41,42,43]. However, epidemiological studies of endemic infective disease are fraught with difficulty.

On the available evidence it seems reasonable to agree with the American Academy of Paediatrics -- "unless carefully controlled clinical studies provide evidence to the contrary, iron fortification of formula and foods seems to provide safe and effective methods for maintaining iron stores and preventing iron deficiency in infancy"[44]. Parenteral iron should rarely if ever be used.

Other non specific protective factors

Human milk contains about 3000 times as much lysozyme as cow's milk. It can be recovered from the faeces of breast-fed but not bottle-fed babies[45]. I am unaware of any studies of the lysozyme content of processed cow's milk and infant formulas.

The lactoperoxidase - thiocyanate - hydrogen peroxide anti-bacterial system may be more important in cow's milk than in human milk. It is most active at low pH and so the buffering effect of milk limits its activity. In the human infant the salivary lacto-peroxidase system may be more effective[46].

However whey, the basis of demineralised whey formulas, contains high levels of lactoperoxidase. No use is made of this at present but it has potentially useful antibacterial qualities. A source of hydrogen peroxide is necessary in the system so it is interesting that lactobacilli produce peroxide and can, therefore, activate it so leading to a substantial reduction in the growth of E. coli[45].

FORMULAS FOR ALLERGIC BABIES

    A variety of formulas may be used in children with allergies
although not all of them have been designed specifically for this
purpose.

Types of formulas and milk

    Breast milk is the best alternative, but if this is unavailable
four types of formula or milk are available.

    (a) Heat treated cow's milk: e.g. evaporated milks.

    (b) Milk of other mammals: e.g. goat's milk.

    (c) Hydrolysed cow's milk protein or synthetic amino acid
         Mixtures: e.g. Nutramigen, Pregestimil, Vivonex, Flexical.

    (d) Substituted whole protein -- usually either soya or meat
         protein: e.g. various soya 'milk' preparations based
         either on soya flour or a soya isolate, comminuted chicken
         mixture, beef or lamb heart.

Two major groups of problems arise in the use of these formulas,
the antigenicity of the protein component, and other qualities of
the formula or milk.

Antigenicity of the protein

    The effect of heat treatment on antigenicity has already been
discussed. There seems no doubt that antigenicity, particularly of
the more heat labile whey proteins, is substantially reduced, but
this reduction is often insufficient for the genetically susceptible
child[47].

    There is some cross reactivity between certain proteins in cow's
milk and goat's milk and this may be why some children with cow's
milk allergy cannot tolerate goat's milk either[48]. Similarly a
proportion of children are sensitive to soya protein[49,50,51] and
circulating antibodies have also been found in animals fed casein
hydrolysate[52].

    It is difficult to unravel the evidence. The presence of
circulating food antibodies does not necessarily implicate allergy
as the primary cause of the disease, nor even does it imply allergy.
It has been said that there are no available immunological tests on
which the diagnosis of milk protein allergy can be based[18].
Furthermore, while the primary allergic reaction may cause intestinal
damage, once the intestine is damaged mucosal permeability will
probably increase and so antibodies may occur to whatever protein
the child is receiving therapeutically.

What is the potential allergenicity of various proteins to a child who, at least initially, has a normal intestine but who for some reason is susceptible to allergic disease? Evidence based on detection of circulating antibodies by a haemagglutination technique suggests that soya protein is at least as antigenic as milk protein and should be used with caution in prophylaxis against dietetically induced allergy. Casein hydrolysate resulted in lower antibody titres[53]. I am unaware of studies of the allergenicity of animal flesh protein as used in chicken, lamb and beef based formulas.

Other problems

(a) Goat's milk. Goat's milk has a high solute load, similar to that of cow's milk, and for the human infant is deficient in folic acid so that megaloblastic anaemia may occur[54].

(b) Soya. Soya in its natural state contains trypsin inhibitors, a goitrogen, and its protein is deficient in sulphur amino acids. However, all of these potential problems can be dealt with in the manufacturing process. Some formulas based on soya flour or soya isolate have proven as nutritionally sound as milk based formulas, but results vary considerably from one product to another[55] so that some caution is necessary. Certainly my own experience with a soya flour preparation in the management of kwashiorkor was unsatisfactory[56] although others[57] using a soya isolate formula achieved a good response.

(c) Lactose content. The available soya formulas and those based on casein hydrolysate are free of lactose. Two bodies advising on the composition of formulas for normal children have advised that lactose should always be present. The European Society of Paediatric Gastroenterology and Nutrition advised that the only carbohydrate present should be lactose[58]. The British Department of Health has recommended that the minimum should be 2 g per 100 ml of feed[59].

(d) Fat blends. A vegetable oil is incorporated in most of the special formulas. Many of the fat blends used have a very high content (30% to 50%) of polyunsaturated fatty acids which will accumulate in body fat. In the presence of an adequate vitamin E intake this accumulation is not known to cause any harm, but concern has been expressed that an excessive amount might inhibit the synthesis of the very long chain derivatives of linolenic acid, and any measure which leads to substantial changes in body composition deserves cautious use. It has been suggested therefore that in formulas for normal children linolenic acid should not exceed 20% of the total fatty acids[59]. Some special formulas sometimes used for the allergic child contain up to 40% of the fat as medium chain triglyceride (e.g. Pregestimil). This is probably metabolised completely and so does not appear in depot fat, but it is an unusual food constituent and its use in most allergic infants is necessary only when they have severe malabsorption.

(e) <u>Osmolality and acid load</u>. The osmolality of hydrolysed
casein formulas is usually high unless this can be balanced by a
reduction in the osmolality of the other constituents e.g. the use
of oligosaccharides such as maltodextrin instead of disaccharides.
There have been problems with the acid load of special formulas such
as Nutramigen[60,61], but this can be partly avoided by the use of
suitable mineral mixtures and it seems less of a problem with more
recent formulations. The osmolality and acid load are even higher
in the 'elemental' formulas containing synthetic mixtures of
individual amino acids, glucose (not glucose polymers) and fat.

The decision to put a child onto a special formula should not,
therefore, be taken lightly. Will it indeed be less allergenic?
Can it be used safely in the particular child? The special formulas
are powerful and, therefore, complex products. They have been
designed with skill and care and they should be used as any drug with
full knowledge of indications, mode of action, necessary monitoring,
and potential complications. When used wisely they are an invaluable
and at times life saving tool.

REFERENCES

1. Gerstenberger H.J. and Ruh H.D. (1915) Am. J. Dis. Child. <u>10</u>:
    247-265.
2. Gerstenberger H.J. and Ruh H.D. (1919) Am. J. Dis. Child. <u>17</u>:
    1-37.
3. Oppe T.E., Arneil G.C., Creery R.D.G., Lloyd J.K., Stroud C.E.,
    Wharton B.A. and Widdowson E.M., "Present Day Practice in
    Infant Feeding", Department of Health and Social Security
    Reports on Health and Social Subjects No. 9, London, HMSO.
4. Wharton B.A. and Berger H.M. (1976) BMJ <u>1</u>: 1326-1331.
5. Bullen C.L. and Willis A.T. (1971) BMJ <u>3</u>: 338-343.
6. Kildeberg P. and Winters R.W. (1978) Advances in Paediatrics
    <u>25</u>: 349-381.
7. Berger H.M., Scott P.H., Kenward C., Scott P. and Wharton B.A.
    (1978) Arch. Dis. Child. <u>53</u>: 926-930.
8. Harrison V.C. and Peat G. (1972) BMJ <u>4</u>: 515-518.
9. Bullen C.L., Tearle P.V. and Willis A.T. (1976) J. Med.
    Microbiol. <u>9</u>: 325-333.
10. Bullen C.L., Tearle P.V. and Willis A.T. (1976) J. Med
    Microbiol. <u>9</u>: 335-244.
11. György P. (1971) Am. J. Clin. Nutr. <u>24</u>: 970-975.
12. Bullen C.L., Tearle P.V. and Stewart M.G. (1977) J. Med.
    Microbiol. <u>10</u>: 403-413.
13. Willis A.T., Bullen C.L., Williams K., Fagg C.G., Bourne A. and
    Vignon M. (1973) BMJ <u>4</u>: 67-72.
14. Reiter B., Brock J.H. and Steel E.D. (1975) Immunology <u>28</u>:
    83-95.
15. Griffiths E. and Humphreys J. (1977) Infection and Immunity <u>15</u>:
    396-401.

16. Hilpert H., Gerber H., Amster H., Pahud J.J., Ballabriga A.,
     Avcalis L., Farriaux F., de Payer E. and Nussle D. (1977)
     "Food and Immunology", Almqrist and Wiksell International,
     Stockholm, pp. 182-196.
17. Ratner B., Dworetzky M, Oguri S. and Ascheim L. (1958)
     Paediatrics 22: 449-452.
18. Lebenthal E. (1975) Pediat. Clin. N. Amer. 22: 827-833.
19. Anderson K.J., McLaughlan P., Devey M.E. and Coombs R.R.A.
     (1979) Clin. Exp. Immunol. 35: 454-461.
20. Saperstein S. and Anderson D.W. (1962) J. Pediat. 61: 196-204.
21. Crawford L.V. (1960) Pediatrics 25: 432-436.
22. Ratner B., Dworetzky M., Oguri S. and Ascheim L. (1958)
     Pediatrics 22: 648-659.
23. Davies W. (1958) Arch. Dis. Child. 33: 265-268.
24. Soothill J.F. (1977) in "Food and Immunology" ed. Hambraeus L.,
     Hanson L.A. and McFarlene H., Almqrist and Wiksell
     International, Stockholm, pp. 88-91.
25. Parish W.E., Barrett A.M., Coombs R.R.A., Gunther M. and
     Camps F.E. (1960) Lancet 2: 1106-1110.
26. Coe J.I. and Peterson R.D.A. (1963) J. Lab. Clin. Med. 62:
     477-481.
27. Biering-Sorensen F., Jorgensen T. and Hilden J. (1978) Acta
     Paediatr. Scand. 67: 129-137.
28. Björksten F. and Saarinen (1978) Lancet 2: 624-625.
29. Coombs R.R.A., Devey M.E. and Anderson K.J. (1977) Clin. Exp.
     Immunol. 32: 263-270.
30. Committee on Nutrition (1976) Pediatrics 58: 765-768.
31. Owen G.M., Lubin A.H. and Garry P.J. (1971) J. Pediatr. 79:
     563-568.
32. Department of Health and SOcial Security, "A nutrition survey
     of preschool children 1967-68", Report on Health and Social
     Subjects 10: 74, London, HMSO.
33. McMillan J.A., Oski F.A., Lourie G., Tomarelli R.M. and
     Landaw S.A. (1977) Pediatrics 60: 896-901.
34. Schade A.L. and Caroline L. (1946) Science 104: 340-342.
35. Bullen J.J., Rogers H.J. and LEigh L. (1972) BMJ 1: 69-75.
36. Scott P.H., Berger H.M., Kenward C., Scott P. and Wharton B.A.
     (1975) Arch. Dis. Child. 50: 796-798.
37. Farmer K. and Becroft D.M.O. (1976) Arch. Dis. Child. 51: 486.
38. Baltimore R.S., Becchilto J.S. and Pearson H.A. (1978)
     Pediatrics 62: 1072-1074.
39. Brozovic B., Burland W.L., Simpson K. and Lord J. (1974) Arch.
     Dis. Child 49: 386-389.
40. Mellhorn D.K. and Gross S. (1971) J. Pediatr. 79: 569-580.
41. Salmi T., Hanninen P. and Peltonen T. (1963) Acta Paediatr.
     Scand. Suppl. suppl. 140: 114-115 (Abst.).
42. Akelman M.B. and Sered B.R. (1966) Am. J. Dis. Child. 111: 45-55.
43. Burman D. (1972) Arch. Dis. Child. 47: 261-271.
44. Committee on Nutrition, "Relationship between iron status and
     incidence of infection in childhood" (1978) Pediatrics 62:
     246-250.

45. Reiter B. (1978) J. Dairy Res. 45: 131-147.
46. Gothefors L. and Marklund S. (1975) Infect. Immun. 11: 1210-1215.
47. Freier S., Kletter B., Gery I. et al. (1969) J. Pediat. 75:
     623-631.
48. Meiner D.C., Sears J.W. and Kniker W.T. (1962) Am. J. Dis. Child.
     103: 634-654.
49. Mendoza J. and Meyers J. (1970) Pediatrics 46: 774-775.
50. Ament M.E. and Rubin C.E. (1972) Gastroenterology 62: 227-234.
51. Whitington P.F. and Gibson R. (1977) Pediatrics 59: 730-732.
52. Seban A., Konijn A.M. and Freier S. (1977) Am. J. Clin. Nutr.
     30: 840-846.
53. Eastham E.J., Liehauco T., Grady M.I. and Wlaker W.A. (1978)
     J. Pediatr. 93: 561-564.
54. Ford J.E. and Scott K.J. (1968) J. Dairy Res. 35: 85-90.
55. Fomon S.J. and Filer L.J. (1974) Soya based formulas in "Infant
     Nutrition" ed. Fomon S.J., Saunders, Philadelphia, pp. 387-390.
56. Rutishauser I.E.H. and Wharton B.A. (1968) Arch. Dis. Child.
     43: 463-467.
57. Graham G.G., Placko R.P., Morales E., Acevedo G. and Cordano A.
     (1970) Am. J. Dis. Child. 120: 419-423.
58. European Society Paediatric Gastroenterology and Nutrition (1977)
     Recommendations for the ocmposition of an adapted formula,
     Acta Paed. Scand. Suppl. 262: 1-20.
59. Department of Health and Social Security. Food for the young
     infant. Report of the Working Party on the Composition of
     Foods for Infants (in press), London, HMSO.
60. Healy C.E. (1972) Pediatrics 49: 910-911.
61. Kildeberg P. and Winters R. (1972) Pediatrics 49: 801-802.

IMMUNOLOGICAL IMPLICATIONS OF ALTERNATIVES TO MOTHER'S MILK

II   DONOR MILK

Brian Wharton

Sorrento and Birmingham Maternity Hospitals
Birmingham
United Kingdom

When a mother for whatever reason does not lactate successfully her baby usually receives an infant formula commonly based on cow's milk. In certain circumstances, however, breast milk from a donor may be given instead. There are three main ways in which donor milk is used. Many neonatal physicians consider that for a pre-term baby donor breast milk is the next best to his mother's own fresh milk particularly during the first week or so of life when the fear of necrotising enterocolitis is greatest. Similarly neonatal surgeons have by experinece adopted donor breast milk as the first choice for babies recovering from operations particularly on the gastrointestinal tract. Finally in severe cases of cow's milk protein intolerance, when there is inanition due to continuing diarrhoea and profound malabsorption, donor breast milk may on occasion save life and be a much safer, simpler, and cheaper alternative to a combination of parenteral nutrition and semi-elemental diets. Donor milk may also be given to a child with a strong family history of atopy but in practice some other alternative is usually used, probably because donor breast milk is so difficult to get that its use must be limited to short periods in babies with potentially lethal problems.

The unique immunological properties of breast milk are well known[1,2,3]. This chapter gives a brief historical background of breast milk donation, describes the activities of the milk bank at Sorrento Maternity Hospital in Birmingham, and discusses the need for and the immunological implications of the various processes currently used in human milk banking.

WET NURSING AND THE EARLY MILK BANKS

Donor breast milk was originally supplied directly to the infant by wet nurses and what was probably the first special care baby unit in the world; Pierre Budin's unit in Paris had a group of formidable donors. He had a panel of resident wet nurses each looking after three or four babies including her own, an average secretion of over 2 litres a day from each wet nurse was sometimes obtained[4].

Ill adults would also use wet nurses and the following description of the use of wet nurses by Dr Caius, the founder of Caius College, is given by Thomas Muffett[5].

> "What made Dr Caius in his last sickness so peevish
> and so full of frets at Cambridge, when he suckt one
> woman (whom I spare to name) froward of conditions
> and of bad diet; and contrariwise so quiet and well,
> when he suckt another of contrary disposition?
> verily the diversity of their milks and conditions,
> which being contrary one to the other, wrought also
> in him that sucked them contrary effects."

Thomas Phaire[6] in the first book on paediatrics ever written by an Englisham was at great pains to describe a suitable wet nurse and the desirable qualities of donor milk.

> "Wherfore as it is agreing to nature so is it also
> necessary & comly for the own mother to nource the
> owne chylde. Whiche if it may be done, it shall be
> moste comendable and holsome, if not ye must be well
> aduised in takyng of a nource, not of ill complexion
> and of worse manners: but suche as shalbe sobre,
> honeste and chaste, well fourmed, amyable and cheare-
> full, so that she may accustome the infant vnto mirth,
> no dronkarde, vicious nor sluttysshe, for suche
> corrupteth the nature of the chylde.
>
> But an honest woman, (such as had a man childe
> last afore) is best not within twoo monethes after
> her delyueraunce, nor approchyng nere vnto her time
> againe. These thynges ought to be cosidered of
> euery wise person, that wyll set their chyldren
> out to nource. Moreouer, it is good to loke vpon
> the milke, and to se whether it be thicke & grosse,
> or to muche thinne and watry, blackysshe or blewe,
> or enclinynge to reddenesse or yelowe, for all
> suche are vnnaturall and euill. Likewyse when ye
> tast it in your mouthe, yf it be eyther bitter,
> salte, or soure, ye may well perceyue it is unhol-
> some.

> That milke is good, that is whyte and sweete,
> and when ye droppe it on your nayle, and do moue
> your finger, neither fleteth abrode at euery stering
> nor will hange faste vpon your nayle, whe ye turne
> it downeward, but that which is betwene both is best."

Wet nursing was disappearing however and by the 18th century the
Governors of the Foundling Hospital were suggesting to the Royal
College of Physicians that 'hand' rearing might be better.

> "First, Whether it will be most prudent for the
> Governors to endeavour to provide Wet Nurses for
> all the Children they take in? or whether it will
> not be better to bring up by hand all such as will
> feed, and suckle only those that will not?
> Second, How Long ought a Child to continue to Suck?" [7]

In 1910 Dr Fritz B. Talbot organised an institution in Boston
which, as well as maintaining a list of suitable wet nurses, began
the systematic collection and distribution of human milk. Adequate
preservation was a problem and the milk had to be used within a few
hours of secretion. In 1922 Emerson[8] reported his first experiments
with preservation of human milk. He found it was possible to preserve
the fat skimmed from the milk and he also experimented with roller
dried breast milk[9] but in 1933 with the help of the Borden milk
company he studied and perfected the process of deep freezing the
milk[10]. By 1931 the Boston "Directory for Mothers Milk" was
collecting 4400 quarts annually and distributing it to 22 hospitals.
They were also at this time pasteurising but it is uncertain exactly
when this was introduced. Other cities followed including Chicago,
New York, Los Angeles, Pittsburgh, Detroit and Montreal. In 1939
the Directory published a set of standards describing all aspects of
human milk banking[11] including pasteurisation and freezing and in
1943 the American Academy of Paediatrics issued national standards,
based mostly on the Boston ones[12].

The human milk bank at Helsinki Children's Hospital began about
fifty years ago. Today it processes over 11,000 litres per year.
Since its inception mothers have left milk at one of a chain of
grocery stores in Helsinki to await collection[13].

The first milk bank in Britain opened at Queen Charlotte's,
London, in 1937. The second world war inhibited the developement of
further banks but following unpublished studies by Walker at the
Willesden and Perivale maternity hospitals the Medical Research
Council, at the request of the Ministry of Health, appointed a small
committee to enquire into the possibility of preparing and
distributing dried human milk. The committee rejected the suggestion
but did commission studies on the bacteriology, sterilisation and
freezing of human milk[15,16,17].

In the immediate post war years a number of hospitals ran banks
for their own use, not aiming to supply other institutions[14,17]
and in addition larger units, modelled on the one at Queen Charlotte's
were opened offering a service to other hospitals as well as their
own. Centres were organised in Cardiff in 1948, Birmingham and
Bristol in 1950 and a little later in Leicester and Liverpool[18].

In 1973 there were five large 'commercial' banks in Britain, at
Queen Charlotte's Lonodn, St David's Cardiff, Sorrento Birmingham,
Southmead Bristol and Royal Alexandra in Brighton, which, apart from
meeting their own requirements, sold processed milk to other institutions. They produced 9000 litres per year and all used pasteurisation
followed by deep freezing[19]. Only two of these banks now regularly
supply other hospitals as well, St David's and Sorrento. In recent
years, however, there has been a renaissance of interest in the value
of human milk and there is now an established service in at least
another fifteen hospitals which collect and process milk for their
own use. The U.K. Department of Health has set up a working party
to advise on the organisation of human milk banks and its report is
awaited.

THE SORRENTO MILK BANK

The initiative for a breast milk bank in Birmingham came from
the Institute of Child Health. It started in 1950 in an eight-roomed
house rented from the Children's Hospital on a site where the present
Institute of Child Health building stands, and it was run by the City
health authorities. In 1955 the bank moved to Sorrento Maternity
Hospital and the organisation was taken over by the hospital[18,20].

Today the bank processes about 1000 litres per year. Most of
it is used withing Birmingham, but about one fifth is sent to other
centres on request within about 150 mile radius. The milk is almost
wholly collected from mothers at home using expression by hand or
hand pump, or by the drip method into a nipple cup. The hand pump
or nipple cup are sterilised with hypochlorite before use, and the
mothers are asked to wash their breasts with ordinary soap and water
before the donation. After collection the milk is poured into a
sterile bottle supplied by the hospital and stored for up to four
days in the 4°C section of the mother's refrigerator.

When donors are first accepted their WR and Australia antigen
serology is checked via their antenatal records and their first
donation of breast milk is examined bacteriologically. About 3% of
these donations contain S. aureus and 15% contain enterobacteria and
collection from these mothers is tactfully stopped.

Once a mother has been accepted to the panel of donors further
individual donations from her are not routinely examined bacteriologically. All milk from the accepted panel of mothers is pooled

pasteurised in 500 ml bottles. The holder system is used, i.e. 65°C
for 30 minutes followed by rapid cooling with time clock control and
automatic temperature chart recording of the process. A test sample
from the pool is processed at the same time and subsequently cultured.
The pasteurised milk is stored at -18°C for up to six months, but
usually for less than two months. Routine monitoring of nutrient
content is not performed but a pooled sample of donations performed
as part of a Department of Health study gave results very similar to
those of other centres and the previously well known composition of
breast milk[21].

     The milk is collected or sent by the rapid parcel service of
British Rail.

WHY HEAT TREAT

     If donor milk could be fed almost immediately to the baby, and
only after contact with sterile vessels, then bacterial contamination
would be little more than for the breast-fed baby and so presumably
treatment would not be necessary.

     Breast milk contains bacteria most of which originate from the
skin of the breast and from a little way into the nipple ducts, and
which are mainly skin organisms such as staphylococcus epidermides
and albus[22,23,24,25], but an appreciable number, particularly
streptococci and sometimes S. aureus, probably originate from the
mouth of the donor's own baby[23,26,27]. Faecal organisms are less
common but do occur and in poor circumstances may be found in large
number, for example in Guatemalan Indian mothers[28].

     This natural and possibly harmless contamination may be made
worse, however, by contamination of collecting vessels, followed by
the opportunity for the organisms to multiply in the time between
collection and consumption.

     Table 1 summarises eleven studies of the bacteriology of breast
milk. They mostly describe milk as it arrived at a milk bank. In
many instances this was up to three days after secretion, during
which time the milk would have been stored in a domestic refrigerator
ostensibly at 4°C but in practice few refrigerators at home maintain
this. The results are variable and sometimes difficult to reconcile,
for example 93% of the Leicester samples had more than 10 organisms
per ml even though they were cultured within an hour of collection
whereas in none of the other studies did this count occur in more
than 50% of the samples even though milk had been delivered to a bank
after a delay. It is possible that many of the organisms died during
the delay, or that the Leicester mothers collected the milk in an
unsatisfactory way, or there may be methodological differences.

Table 1. Bacteriology of untreated human milk arriving in banks (except No. 9) from mothers at home or in hospital.

Method of collection	Number studied	Mean count	Bacterial counts per ml						Centre and reference
			All organisms % donations with counts shown				Potential pathogens % donations and count		
			Sterile	$1{-}10^3$	$10^3{-}10^6$	$>10^6$	S. aureus	Enterobacteria	
1. Manual expression Hand pump	152	2500							Stamford, California[29]
	43	10^5							
2. Home and hospital, expressed	59						37	54 'coliforms' 9 E. coli	Szeged, Hungary[30]
3. Manual or pump expression	2093		56	4	25	15	1 (10^7)	5 (10^7)	Whipps Cross, London[31]
4. Most manual or hand pump. Some drip. Hypochlorite sterilisation of collecting vessels.	371		59		35	6	1	8	Kings College Hospital, London[32,33]
5. As 4. As above but rejecting first 10 ml.	355		54		41	5	5	33 all lactose fermenters	(25)
	172		79		20	1	1	9	
6. Drip	6 pools	10^7					a 17 (10^6)	51 (10^6)	Oxford, England[34]
Drip with hypochlorite sterilisation of vessels	6 pools	$10^{5.5}$					17 (10^5)	34 (10^5)	
7. Manual expression at home	175		(<2500) 67	(2.5-5000) 9		(>5000) 23	3 (10^3)	18 (10^3)	Fazakerley Hospital, Liverpool[35]
Mainly pump in hospital	513		67	10		23	4 (10^3)	4 (10^3)	
8. Manual expression first 5 ml.	20	3500							Stamford, California (36)
Manual expression rejection first 5 ml.	20	700							
9. Drip. Cultured within 1 hr.	207		3	5	87	5	a 6 (10^8)	7 (10^7)	Leicester, England[37]
10. Manual expression into domestic vessels.	14 pools				42	58			London, England[38]
Manual expression into autoclaved bottles	15 pools		87		13		18	10	
11. Home collections	1075		49	(1-10^4) 38		(>10^4) 13			Tampere, Finland[39]

a Group B streptococci found in a few instances.

The table does indicate useful points of technique in milk collection to minimise the bacterial count. It seems an advantage to use collecting and storage vessels either sterilised by autoclaving or after soaking in hypochlorite. Hand pumps often increase contamination because it is very difficult to sterilise the rubber bulb. The first 5 to 10 ml expressed should be discarded because this milk 'washes out' the duct exits and also the areola and so contains more bacteria.

Notions of what constitutes a 'safe' count, however, are quite arbitrary and indeed it is difficult to suggest a protocol which would establish the upper limit of a safe bacterial count. The views of various authorities are shown in Table 2, but since all of the babies in the Leicester study (Table 1) thrived despite the higher counts found, perhaps these counts even though they are much higher than the limits in Table 2 are acceptable so long as the 'protective' factors present in breast milk remain intact. On the other hand definite examples of Salmonella and Group B streptococcal infection from human milk have been described[41,42,43].

The authorities quoted in Table 2 all feed milk which has not been heated (deep frozen and rethawed if necessary) if it achieves their chosen criteria. At Sorrento we pasteurise all milk irrespective of the count and examine a sample bacteriologically afterwards. Some centres reject milk even for pasteurisation unless it fulfils certain criteria (Table 2). As far as I am aware there have been no similar systematic studies of viruses in human milk although hepatitis B virus, cytomegalvirus and rubella virus have been found in human milk[44,45,46].

THE EFFECTS OF HEAT TREATMENT

If milk is heated to reduce its bacterial count what does this do to the various protective factors? Boiling is very destructive but holder pasteurisation (65°C for 30 minutes) achieves a substantial reduction in bacterial numbers without complete destruction of the factors. Table 3 summarises six studies of the effects of holder pasteurisation. Some of the studies used a laboratory pasteurisation method and the conditions were probably more carefully controlled than in the average milk bank; the Cardiff study[50] showed that their pasteurisation process in routine use reached 73°C for 30 minutes rather than the intended 65°C. A further caveat is that most of the assessments used were in vitro quantitative biochemical measurements. In only a few instances, for example the Shinfield and Oxford studies[47,48], were any functional effects on bacterial growth included. Only the Edinburgh study examined qualitative as well as quantitative changes.

Table 2. Suggested criteria for feeding untreated, or for pasteurising human milk.

Criteria for feeding untreated milk				Criteria for pasteurisation		Reference
Maximum permitted count of organisms per ml			Proportion of donations which were acceptable on these criteria	Maximum permitted count of organisms before accepted for pasteurisation		
All bacteria	S. aureus	Entero-bacteria		Potential pathogens	All bacteria	
10^4	4×10^3	Nil	90% – 95%			(13)
10^4						(40), (36)
5×10^3	Nil	Nil	71% hospital 55% home	No S. aureus or faecal organisms permitted	5×10^3	(35)
						.
2.5×10^3	10^2	Nil	80% if first 10 ml rejected	S. aureus 10^3	10^5	(32, 33), (25)
2.5×10^3	Nil	Nil	? 60%	Any S. aureus Pseudomonas Klebsiella, etc.	10^6	(31)
Nil			49%		2×10^4	(39)

Table 3. Reduction in protective factors of breast milk following processing (results are reductions expressed as % of level in untreated milk)

Process	Rank?	Holder Pasteurisation 62.5°C for 30 minutes					Deep Frozen			Lyophilised[e]		Gamma irradiation
Nature of pasteurisation	Rank?	Laboratory	Oxford pasteurised	Laboratory	Laboratory	Laboratory						
Number of treated samples[b]	?	1-3 samples from 1 pool	4-11	15	23	6-9	4-11	23	8-16	8-16	23	11
Lactoferrin	65			Nil (+117-37)		57						28(0-80)[d]
Unsaturated iron binding capacity		76							+2	+9		
IgA	22		21	14(+11-44)	33	Nil	1	15	3	2	30	18(0-32)[d]
Antibody to E. coli	0-56			Max 20	50			Nil			20	65
IgG					50	34		50		21	70	
IgM		100			30						80	
C3									7		3	
Lysozyme	Nil		36			24[a]	Nil		10	6		
α1 antitrypsin									17	7		
Cyancobalamin binding capacity		48[c]										
Folic acid binding capacity		10[c]										
Macrophazes		22			100		Nil					
Lymphocytes						100		63% @ 1 wk. 100% @ 2 wks.			100	
Increase in multiplication of E. coli at 3 hours log 10		4.3 to 5.0 / 4.2 to 4.9	4 to 4.5 / 5.2 to 5.3									
Reference	(30)	(47)	(48)	(49)	(40)	(50)	(48)	(40)	(50)	(40)	(50)	(49)

Note: Reductions of less than 15% were mostly not significant by the methods used.
(a) 99% loss at pH7, 27% loss at pH6.
(b) in some papers many more results on untreated samples are presented.
(c) effects on bacterial growth are given.
(d) partially denatured.
(e) see also text re studies of Liebe and Heyde[53].

Nevertheless it seems that after efficient pasteurisation breast milk still maintains a reasonable content of certain protective factors both as measured chemically and by the effects on bacterial growth in vitro. There are few studies of the specific antiviral factors but it seems the non-immunoglobulin macromolecule of Matthews et al resists mild heat treatment and the lipid mediated antiviral activity resists boiling[51,52].

OTHER TREATMENTS

The major alternative to heat treatment is to store at -18°C and thaw immediately before feeding, (Table 2 and Table 3). The number of samples is small but deep freezing seems to have very little effect on the chemical protective factors. Gamma irradiation and freeze drying have also been studied (Table 3) and their adverse effects were small, but gamma irradiation partially denatured IgA and lactoferrin. Freeze drying is used fairly extensively in Germany[53]. About three quarters of the living bacteria are killed by freeze drying and most of the remainder are killed after six weeks' storage so long as the humidity remains less than 4%. Inhibitory qualities against S. corynebacteria, streptococci and mostly against S. aureus were maintained even after two years' storage, but the cost is high, about 180 marks per litre.

If the antibacterial lactoperoxidase system in cow's milk is activated by providing peroxide from added glucose and glucose oxidase it is possible to extend the storage period of raw cow's milk without deterioration due to bacterial growth[54]. Whether this could be adopted in human milk technology is speculative.

THE FUTURE

It is possible that new formulas may resemble more closely the humoral protective qualities of breast milk and so reduce our present reliance on donor milk. In the meantime many paediatricians will rely during critical periods on donor milk; some will be prepared to feed it untreated[31,32], many will pasteurise their own supply perhaps using the convenient Oxford pasteuriser[48], others will rely on supplies from a few remaining central banks.

But what of the cells in fresh human milk? As the flux of immunological interest moves from humoral to cellular factors in breast milk it may be that attention will turn to methods of preserving the cells intact. Nothing is more distressing to the neonatal physician than the loss from necrotising enterocolitis of a baby who was beginning to recover from life threatening respiratory failure. There are almost certainly other factors as well as infection in the aetiology of neonatal necrotising enterocolitis such as asphyxia, ischaemia and some iatrogenic factor. Nevertheless the observation that milk cells protected the newborn rat from experimentally produced enterocolitis[55] supports the clinical observation that enterocolitis is rare (but not unknown) in breast-fed babies. It may be this condition and these observations that will stimulate the next phase in human milk banking: can the cells in donor milk be preserved functionally intact and is it desirable to do so?

REFERENCES

1.   Reiter B. (1978) J. Dairy Res. 45: 131-147.
2.   Pittard W.B. (1979) Am. J. Dis. Child. 133: 83-87.
3.   Welsh J.K. and May J.T. (1978) J. Pediatr. 94: 1-9.
4.   Budin P. (1907) "The Nursling", translation by Maloney W.J., Caxton Publishing Compnany, London, pp. 166-172.
5.   Muffett T. (1655) "Healths Improvement". Quoted by Drummond J.C. and Wilbraham A. (1958) in "The Englishman's Food", Jonathan Cape, London, p. 124.
6.   Phaire T. "The Boke of Chyldren", reprint (1965) E. and S. Livingstone Ltd, Edinburgh and London, pp. 18-19.
7.   Nichols R.H. and Wray F.A. (1935) "The History of the Foundling Hospital". Quoted by Drummond J.C. and Wilbraham A. (1958) in "The Englishman's Food", Jonathan Cape, London, p. 245.
8.   Emmerson P.W. (1922) JAMA 78: 641-642.
9.   Emmerson P.W. and Smith L.W. (1926) Am. J. Dis. Child. 31: 1-21.
10. Emmerson P.W. and Platt W. (1933) J. Pediatr. 33: 472-477.
11. McPherson C.H. and Talbot F.B. (1939) J. Pediatr. 15: 461-468.
12. American Academy of Pediatrics Committee on mothers milk. Recommended standards for the operation of mothers milk bureau. (1943) J. Pediatr. 23: 112-128.
13. Siimes M.M. and Hallman N. (1979) J. Pediatr. 94: 173-174.
14. Dynski-Klein M. (1946) BMJ 2: 258-260.
15. Medical Research Council (1947) "Medical Research in War", London, HMSO, pp. 130, 420.
16. Wright J. (1947) Lancet 2: 121-124.
17. Wright J. and Edwards E.M.C. (1947) Lancet 2: 233-234.
18. Gant L. (1959) Nursing Mirror 24 October iii-iv.
19. Rolles C. (1973) Midwives Chron. 86: 353-354.
20. Mackintosh J.M. (1951) 13 July i-iv.
21. Department of Health and Social Security, "Composition of Human Milk", Report on Health and Social Subjects No. 12, London, HMSO.
22. Foster W.D. and Harris R.E. (1960) J. Obstet. Gynecol. Brit. Emp. 67: 463-464.
23. Plueckhahn V.D. and Banks J. (1964) BMJ 2: 414-418.
24. Gavin A. and Ostovar K. (1979) J. Food Protection 40: 614-616.
25. West P.A., Hewitt J.H. and Murphy O.M. (1979) J. App. Bacteriol. 46: 269-277.
26. Wysham D.N., Mulhern M.E., Nararre G.C., La Veck G.D., Kennan A.L. and Giedt W.R. (1957) New Eng. J. Med. 257: 304-306.

27. McCarthy C., Snyder M.L. and Parker R.B. (1965) Arch. Oral
         Biol. 10: 61-70.
28. Wyatt R.G. and Mata L.J. (1969) J. Trop. Pediatr. 15: 159-162.
29. Liebhaber M., Lewiston N.J., Asquith M.T. and Sunshine P. (1978)
         J. Pediatr. 92: 236-237.
30. Szöllösy E., Marjai E. and Lantos J. (1974) Acta Microbiol.
         Acad. Sci. Hung. 21: 319-325.
31. McEnery G. and Chattopadhyay B. (1978) BMJ 2: 794-796.
32. Williamson S., Hewitt J.H., Finucane E. and Gamsu H.R. (1978)
         BMJ 1: 393-396.
33. Williamson S., Finucane E., Gamsu H.R. and Hewitt J.H. (1978)
         BMJ 1: 1146.
34. Lucas A. and Roberts C.D. (1979) BMJ 1: 80-82.
35. Davidson D.C., Poll R.A. and Roberts C. (1979) Arch. Dis.
         Child. 54: 760-764.
36. Asquith M.T. and Harrod J.R. (1979) J. Pediatr. 6: 993-994.
37. Carroll L., Davies D.P., Osman M. and McNeish A.S. (1979)
         Lancet 2: 732-733.
38. Wright J. (1947) Lancet 2: 121-124.
39. Ikonen R.S. and Maki K. (1977) BMJ 2: 386-387.
40. Liebhaber M., Lewiston N.J., Asquith M.T., Olds-Arrgyo L. and
         Sunshine P. (1977) J. Pediatr. 91: 897-900.
41. Ryder R.W., Crosby-Ritchie A., McDonough B. and Hall W.J. (1977)
         JAMA 238: 1533-1534.
42. Kenny J.F. and Zedd A.J. (1977) J. Pediatr. 91: 158-159.
43. Centre for disease control (1971) "Salmonella Kottbus Meningitis
         associated with contaminated breast milk", Mortality Morbidity
         Weekly Rep. 20: 154.
44. Linnemann C.C. Jr. and Goldberg S. (1974) Lancet 2: 155.
45. Hayes K., Danks D.M., Gibas H. and Jack I. (1972) New Eng. J.
         Med. 287: 157.
46. Emödi G. and Just M. (1974) Scand. J. Immunol. 3: 157.
47. Ford J.E., Law B.A., Marshall V.M.E. and Relter B. (1977) J.
         Pediatr. 90: 29-35.
48. Gibbs J.H., Fisher C., Bhattacharya S., Goddard P. and Baum J.D.
         (1977) Early Human Development 1: 227-245.
49. Raptopoulou-Gigi M., Marwick I. and McClelland D.B.L. (1977)
         BMJ 1: 12-14.
50. Evans T.J., Ryley H.C., Neale L.M., Dodge J.A. and Lewarne V.M.
         (1978) Arch. Dis. Child. 53: 239-241.
51. Mathews T.H.J., Nair C.O.G., Lawrence M.K. and Turell D.A.J.
         (1976) Lancet 2: 1387-1389.
52. Welsh J.K., Skurrie I.J. and May J.T. (1978) Infect. Immun.
         19: 395-401.
53. Liebe von S. and Heyde S. (1969) Dtsch. Gesundheitsw. 24: 170-175.
54. Björck L., Rosen C.G., Marshall V.M.E. and Reiter B. (1975)
         Applied Microbiology 30: 199-204.
55. Pitt J., Barlow B. and Heird W.C. (1977) Pediatric Research
         11: 906-909.

ACKNOWLEDGEMENTS

    I am grateful to Mrs E. Proctor, Sister in Charge of the Sorrento
Milk Bank for her advice; Dr J.G. Bissenden for German translation;
the Medical Illustration Department of the Birmingham Children's
Hospital for the figures, and Mrs P. Cox and Miss P. Morris for
preparing the manuscripts.

IMPLICATIONS FOR IMMUNISATION:

THE MILK IgA ANTIBODY RESPONSE TO LIVE

AND INACTIVATED POLIO VIRUS VACCINES

L.Å. Hanson, B. Carlsson, F. Jalil, B.S. Lindblad
and A-M. Svennerholm

Institute of Medical Microbiology and
Department of Pediatrics
University of Göteborg, Sweden

Department of Social and Preventive Pediatrics
King Edward Medical College, Lahore, Pakistan

Department of Pediatrics of the Karolinska Institute
at St. Göran's Hospital, Stockholm, Sweden

Human milk is rich in secretory IgA (SIgA) antibodies, many of
which are directed against food proteins and antigens of microorganisms found in the intestine[1,2,3]. The appearance of these
milk antibodies against antigens from the intestinal content is
explained by the enteromammaric link: antigenic exposure of the
Peyer's patches leads to homing of cells committed to IgA sunthesis
to various exocrine glands, including the mammary gland[4,5]. In
addition there may be a selective transfer via serum or IgA dimer-J
chain complexes that are taken up by secretory component (SC). The
SC which is produced in epithelial cells in exocrine glands functions
as a receptor on the cell membrane of these epithelial cells. SIgA
is formed by the binding of IgA-J to the SC and is transferred into
the exocrine secretion. At least in mice this serum transfer may
provide a substantial portion of the milk SIgA[6, Halsey personal
communication). Presumably the serum IgA dimers originate from the
extensive production of IgA in the intestinal lamina propria.

In accordance with the function of the enteromammaric link
intestinal antigen exposure results in the appearance of milk antibodies in several species, including man[7,8,9,10,11,3,12,13]. In
the pig intramammary immunisation with a transmissible gastroenteritis

virus primarily induces IgG antibody production as does parenteral
immunisation[14]. Higher and more persistent milk IgA antibody
levels result from peroral immunisation[13]. In the rabbit intramammary immunisation also gives mostly IgG antibodies in milk, but
when Freund's complete adjuvant was used higher milk IgA responses
were formed in those immunised in the mammary gland than when the
antigen was given intrabronchially or intragastrically[10].

      There are few studies of the milk SIgA response in relation to
vaccination in the human. Intestinal colonisation in late pregnancy
with an innocuous E. coli strain[11] as well as with a live Shigella
vaccine[3, Carlsson et al unpublished results) was followed by
specific SIgA antibodies appearing in the milk. Furthermore, we
noticed that subcutaneous immunisation with a killed whole cell
V. cholerae vaccine, besides the expected serum antibody increase,
also resulted in a booster of milk and saliva SIgA antibodies against
the V. cholerae lipopolysaccharide[14]. This study was performed in
Pakistani women who already had SIgA antibodies, presumably as a
result of natural intestinal exposure. In contrast, Swedish women
without previous exposure to V. cholerae and without prevaccination
SIgA antibodies against the V. cholerae antigen did not produce SIgA
antibodies in milk, although there was a serum antibody response[3,
15]. In a recent investigation lactating mothers in Bangladesh were
also found to respond to a cholera toxoid vaccine given parenterally
with milk SIgA antibody formation[16]. These findings suggest that
parenteral immunisation can boost an SIgA response present as a
result of previous intestinal antigen exposure. In consequence
vaccination in endemic areas may enhance not only serum but also
secretory antibodies.

      In order to compare the induction of the milk SIgA antibody
response by peroral and parenteral antigen administration we decided
to employ a perorally given live (LPV) polio virus vaccine and a
parenterally administered inactivated poliovirus (IPV) vaccine in
endemically and non-endemically exposed mothers.

MATERIAL AND METHODS

Lactating women

      Well nourished and healthy Swedish women who had received three
to six subcutaneous (s.c.) doses of IPV during childhood were
immunised with IPV. Undernourished Pakistani women in fairly good
health who had not been vaccinated and had not knowingly had polio
were immunised with either IPV or LPV.

Vaccines

      The Swedish women were given one s.c. dose of 1.0 ml killed
trivalent polio virus vaccine produced by the Swedish National

Bacteriological Laboratory (SBL), Solna, Sweden. The Pakistani
mothers were given 1.0 ml s.c. of the SBL IPV vaccine, or 3 drops
perorally (p.o.) or a live trivalent vaccine from either Institut
Mérieux, Lyon (IML), France, or Connaught Labs Ltd, Toronto, Canada.

Samples

   Milk and in some instances saliva and serum were sampled
immediately before and at two and occasionally four and six weeks
after the immunisation. All samples were obtained in glass vials
by manual expression and immediately frozen at $-20^{\circ}C$. They were
also transported at $-20^{\circ}C$. The milk samples were centrifuged at
4000 x g for 15 minutes using the clear middle layer for titration.

Polio ELISA

   The enzyme-linked immunosorbent assay (ELISA) was adapted for
the polio virus antibody studies as recently described[16]. In these
preliminary studies antigen of polio virus type 1 was prepared from
the Chat Strain, but in the most recent work we used polio antigen
types 1 and 3 kindly provided by Dr van Wezel, Rijks Institut voor
de Volksgesondheid, Bilthoven, Holland. Alkaline-phosphatase-
conjugated antisera against IgG, IgA, IgM and secretory component
(SC) were used to titrate the polio virus antibody levels.

   The titres given are means of 2 to 5 determinations and represent
the inverse of the interpolated dilutions giving an absorbance of
0.4 above background using a 100 minute reaction time for the enzyme
and substrate.

RESULTS

Inactivated polio virus vaccine given parenterally

   The Swedish women had no prevaccination titres in milk and
responded to the IPV with only a low level and temporary appearance
of milk IgA antibodies to polio virus type 1 (Fig. 1). They showed
a booster of their pre-existing serum antibodies. The increase was
primarily confined to the IgG class.

   In a preliminary study the administration of IPV to the Pakistani
women resulted in significant milk IgA antibody responses to polio
virus type 1 in 5/11 (Fig. 1). In two instances the titre decreased.
Continued studies confirmed that pre-existing milk IgA antibodies
resulting from natural exposure could be boosted by parenteral
vaccination. Against polio virus type 1, for instance, the titre
increased in eight of thirteen mothers after two s.c. doses of IPV
and after one dose in four of thirteen. For antibodies to polio
type 3 virus the titre increased after two s.c. doses in eight of
nine mothers (Table 1).

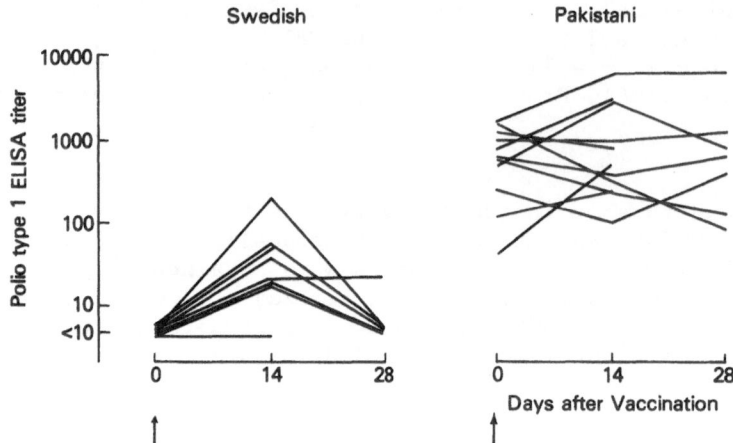

Fig. 1.   Milk IgA antibodies against polio virus type 1 in lactating
Swedish and Pakistani mothers after one SC dose of
inactivated polio virus vaccine.   Arrows indicate
vaccination.

Table 1.   Number of mothers with significant (⩾2 fold) milk Iga antibody response to two subcutaneous doses of inactivated
polio virus vaccine (2 to 6 weeks after vaccination).

Polio virus type	Number of mothers	Milk IgA antibody		
		increase	no change	decrease
1	13	8	5	0
3	9	8	1	0

Peroral immunisation with live poliovirus vaccine

One group of Pakistani women whose milk and saliva IgA antibodies
were boosted by parenteral cholera vaccination[15], was also given
LPV perorally.   A striking decrease was seen in the milk IgA anti-
polio virus type 1 in those who had prevaccination titres (fig. 2).
The decrease was confined to SC-carrying IgA antibodies.   There was
no effect on the low or insignificant milk IgM and IgG antibodies.
In serum there was also no effect on the prevaccination serum IgM
and IgG antibodies, but the serum IgA titres diminished.

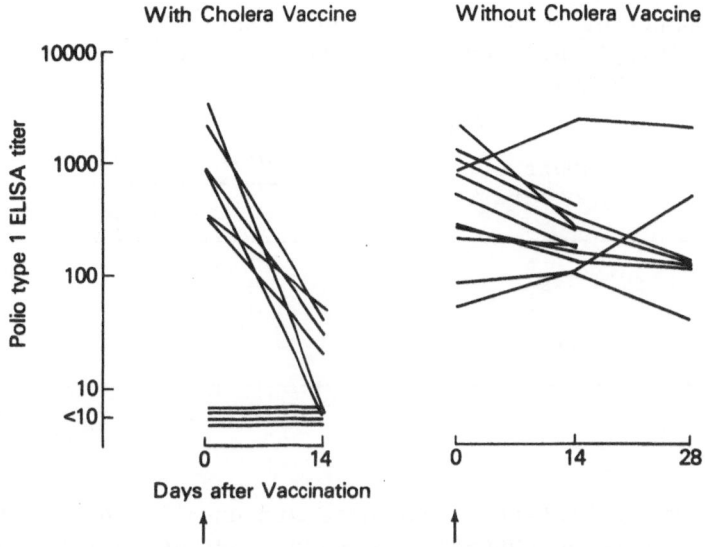

Fig. 2. Milk IgA antibodies against polio virus type 1 in Pakistani
         mothers given live polio virus vaccine perorally either
         alone or simultaneously with one SC dose of cholera vaccine.
         Arrows indicate vaccination.

     The drastic decrease of the milk IgA antibodies seemed partly
to be connected with the simultaneous cholera vaccination since in
a study when LPV was given alone only a titre decrease of smaller
magnitude was found in six of eleven and an increase in two of
eleven of milk IgA anti-polio virus type 1 antibodies (Fig. 2).
The tires continued to decrease over the four week observation period.

     In further investigations it was also seen that the oral LPV
decreased the milk IgA anti-polio virus type 1 antibodies in three
of nine mothers. A significant increase was only seen in one of
nine (Table 2). Antibodies to polio virus type 3 decreased in six
of fourteen cases and showed an increase in three of fourteen
instances.

     Parallel determinations of the milk antibody responses to s.c.
IPV and p.o. LPV with anti-IgA and anti-SC supported our previous
findings[16] that the polio virus antibodies were practically
exclusively of the secretory IgA type.

Table 2. Number of mothers with significant (≥2 fold) changes of
          milk IgA antibody levels after one peroral dose of live
          polio virus vaccine (2 to 4 weeks after vaccination).

Polio virus type	Number of mothers	Milk IgA antibody		
		increase	no change	decrease
1	9	1	5	3
3	14	3	5	6

DISCUSSION

Secretory IgA antibody responses are usually the result of
antigenic exposure on mucosal membranes. Secondary responses can
be induced[17,18,10], but may require repeated doses[19].

In our studies of human milk antibodies it was a striking
finding that in individuals who had prevaccination milk SIgA antibody titres due to natural exposure to V. cholerae or polio virus
a booster was obtained by parenteral vaccination[14,16]. In the
Swedish mothers without such previous encounters there was none or
only a small and temporary increase of milk SIgA antibodies to the
parenteral vaccination[3,15,16]. Further studies are required to
determine whether or not more consistent and higher titre increases
can be obtained with other doses or different spacing of doses.

The finding that the live polio virus vaccine given perorally
in several cases decreased the serum and milk IgA titres was surprising. The mechanism behind this is unclear, but may be related
to the tolerance shown in animal models to peroral antigen exposure
probably caused by the appearance of T suppressor cells specific for
IgA antibody formation[20,21].

It has been claimed that breast milk with high polio virus
antibody titres may interfere with peroral vaccination using LPV[22].
Such a virus neutralisation would agree with the suggested protective
capacity of SIgA antibodies against i.a. certain rhino- and myxovirus
infections[23,24]. Milk SIgA antibodies could in fact be a significant part of the intestinal immunity against polio virus, induced
not only by natural infection but also by vaccination with LPV[25].
It seems that p.o. vaccination of the breast-fed baby with LPV after
several weeks of lactation decreases the risk for interference
between the milk antibodies and the LPV, probably due to the lower
levels of SIgA in mature milk[26,27,28]. Montefiore et al[29]

reported that no interference was seen due to lack of milk antibodies
to polio virus in milk samples from Nigeria. This finding could be
due to a low sensitivity of the method.

In view of the present extensive use of LPV it seems important
to analyse further the mechanisms involved in the decreased milk
SIgA antibodies after peroral live poliovirus vaccination. The poor
efficacy of LPV reported from a number of developing countries[27]
could at least partly be explained by this phenomenon if the milk
IgA antibody response really reflects the intestinal SIgA response.
The booster effect on the milk SIgA antibodies by parenteral
vaccination suggests the possibility to direct and enhance the
immunity provided breast-fed babies via the milk.

ACKNOWLEDGEMENT

These studies were supported by grants from the Swedish Medical
Research Council (Nos. 215 and 3382), SAREC and the Ellen, Walter
and Lennart Hesselman Foundation for Scientific Research.

L. Hanson was an International Fogarty Center Scholar-in-
Residence at the National Institutes of Health, U.S.A., from
August 1979 to September 1980.

REFERENCES

1. Gindrat J-J., Gothefors L., Hanson L.Å. and Winberg J. (1972)
       Acta Paediatr. Scand. 61: 587-590.
2. Holmgren J., Hanson L.Å., Carlsson B., Lindlad B.S. and
       Rahimtoola J. (1976) Scand. J. Immunol. 5: 867-871.
3. Hanson L.Å., Carlsson B., Cruz J.R., Garcia B., Holmgren J.,
       Shaukat R. Khan, Lindlad B.S., Svennerholm A-M.,
       Svennerholm B. and Urrutia J.J. (1979) in "Immunology of
       Breast Milk", Ogra P.L. and Dayton D. eds., Raven Press,
       New York, p. 145.
4. Lamm M.E., Weisz-Carrington P., Roux E., McWilliams M. and
       Phillips-Quagliata J.M. (1979) in "Immunology of Breast
       Milk", Ogra P.L. and Dayton D. eds., Raven Press, New York,
       p. 105.
5. Bienenstock J., McDermott M. and Befus D. (1979) in "Immunology
       of Breast Milk", Ogra P.L. and Dayton D. eds., Raven Press,
       New York, p. 91.
6. Halsey J., Johnson B.H. and Cebra J. (1980) J. Exp. Med. 151:
       767-772.
7. Porter P., Noakes D.E. and Allen W.D. (1970) Immunology 18:
       245-257.
8. Bohl E.H., Gupta R.P.K., Olquin F.M.W. and Saif L.J. (1972)
       Infect. Immun. 6: 289-301; Bohl E.H. and Saif L.J. (1975)
       Infect Immun. 11: 23-32.

9. Montgomery P.C., Cohn J. and Lally E.T. (1974) in "The Immuno-
    globulin A System", Mestecky J. and Lawton A.R. eds., Plenum
    Press, New York, p. 453.
10. Montgomery P.C., Cohen C., Skandera C.A. and Connelly K.M.
    (1979) in " "Immunology of Breast Milk" Ogra P.L. and
    Dayton D. eds., Raven Press, New York, p. 115.
11. Goldblum R.M., Ahlstedt S., Carlsson B., Hanson L.Å., Jodal U.,
    Lidin-Janson G. and Sohl-Åkerlund A. (1975) Nature 257:
    797-799.
12. Porter P. and Chidlow J.W. (1979) in "Immunology of Breast Milk",
    Ogra P.L. and Dayton D. eds., Raven Press, New York, p. 49.
13. Saif L.J. and Bohl E.H. (1979) in "Immunology of Breast Milk",
    Ogra P.L. and Dayton D. eds., Raven Press, New York, p. 237.
14. Svennerholm A-M, Holmgren J., Hanson L.Å., Lindblad B.S.,
    Quereshi F. and Rahimtoola J. (1977) Scand. J. Immunol. 6:
    1345-1349.
15. Svennerholm A-M., Hanson L.Å., Holmgren J., Lindblad B.S.,
    Nilsson B. and Quereshi F. (1980) Infect. Immun. (in press).
16. Svennerholm A M., Hanson L.Å., Svennerholm B., Holmgren J.,
    Lindblad B.S. and Shaukat R. Kahn (1981) J. Infect. Dis.
    (in press).
17. Pierce N.F. and Gowans J.L. (1975) J. Exp. Med. 142: 1550-1563.
18. Pierce N.F. (1978) J. Exp. Med. 148: 195-206.
19. Lange S. and Holmgren J. (1978) Acta Path. Microbiol. Scand.,
    Sect. C 86: 145-152.
20. Elson C.O., Heck J.A. and Strober W. (1979) J. Exp. Med. 149:
    632-641.
21. Richman L.K. (1979) in "Immunology of Breast Milk", Ogra P.L.
    and Dayton D. eds., Raven Press, New York, p. 49; Sabin A.B.
    (1980) Bull. WHO 58: 141-157.
22. Warren R.J., Lepow M.L., Bartsch G.E. and Robbins F.C. (1964)
    Pediatrics 34: 4-13.
23. Smith C.B., Purcell R.H., Bellanti J.A. and Chanock R.M. (1966)
    New Eng. J. Med. 275: 1145-1152.
24. Perkins J.C., Knopf H.L.S., Kapikian A.Z. and Chanock R.M.
    (1971) in "The Secretory Immunologic System", Dayton D.,
    Small P.A., Chanock R.M., Kaufman H.E. and Tomasi T.B. eds.,
    U.S. Dept. of Health, Education and Welfare, NIH, Bethesda,
    p. 203.
25. Ogra P.L. and Carzon D.T. (1969) J. Immunol. 102: 1423-1431.
26. Deforest A., Parker P.B., Di Liberti J.H., Yates H.T. Jr.,
    Sikinga M.S. and Smith D.S. (1973) Pediatrics 83: 93-95.
27. Dömök I., Balayan M.S., Fayinka O.A., Škrtić N., Soneji A.D.
    and Harland P.S.E.G. (1974) Bull. WHO 51: 333-347.
28. John T.J., Devarajan L.V., Luther L. and Vijagarathman P.
    (1976) Pediatrics 57: 47-53.
29. Montefiore D., Collard P., Jamieson M.F. and Jolly H. (1963)
    BMJ II 1569-1572.

INDEX

Acetate buffer in breast or
  bottle-fed in infants,
  44-45, 51-52
Acid load in special formulas,
  120
Allergic babies, formulas for,
  118-120
Allergy, food *see* Food allergy
Anaphylactic sensitivity, 17
Antibody(ies)
  affinity
    in chronic antigen-antibody
      complex disease, 98-99
      effect of human serum
        albumin, 102
      in protein deprivation, 102
    relationship to malnutrition,
      97-106
    effects, 100
  antiviral, in milk, 56-59
  lymphocytes action, 58
  plaque counts, 57
  in bacterial inhibition of
    milk, 35
  circulating, to food proteins,
    19
  to cow's milk protein, 19
Antigen-antibody complex disease
  chronic, effect of protein
    deprivation, 102-104
  effects of malnutrition,
    101-104
  and genetically-control and
    immunodeficiency, 98-99
  induction, in low and high
    affinity, 100-101, 102
  macrophage function, 99

Antigen-antibody complex disease
    (continued)
  role of antibody affinity, 98-99
Antigen(s)
  cow's milk, detection in infant's
    serum, 14-15
  exclusion, mechanism, 16-17
  exposure, early and tolerance in
    suckling, 71
    in animals of immunised
      mothers, 76-78
    older animals, lgE response
      suppression, 72-75
  food, *see* Food antigens
  ingested, handling, 13-22
    allergies, 18
    antifood antibodies, 15
    atopic allergy, 18
    circulating antibodies, 17, 19
    enzyme activity, 16
    factors controlling absorption,
      15-16
    immune exclusion, 16-17
    immune interaction phenomena,
      17-18
    role of Peyer's patches, 18
Antiviral antibodies in milk, 56-58
  lymphocytes, action, 58
  other antiviral substances, 57-59
  plaque counts, 57
Asthma
  and eczema, association, 66-67
  frequency in late autumn birth, 66
Atopic
  allergy and ingested antigens, 18
    and breast feeding, 18
  eczema, 68